ULTRA-PROCESSED FOODS

Concerns, Controversies, and Exceptions

MICHAEL GREGER, M.D., FACLM

New York Times Bestselling Author of *How Not to Die,*
How Not to Diet, and *How Not to Age*

Founder of NutritionFacts.org

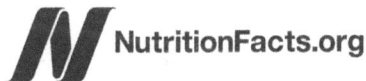

Ɱ NutritionFacts.org

Also by Michael Greger, M.D., FACLM

How Not to Die

The How Not to Die Cookbook

How Not to Diet

The How Not to Diet Cookbook

How to Survive a Pandemic

How Not to Age

The How Not to Age Cookbook

Ozempic: Risks, Benefits, and Natural Alternatives to GLP-1 Weight-Loss Drugs

Lower LDL Cholesterol Naturally with Food

This book contains the opinions and ideas of its author. It is intended to provide helpful general information on the subjects that it addresses. It is not in any way a substitute for the advice of the reader's own physician(s) or other medical professionals based on the reader's own individual conditions, symptoms, or concerns. If the reader needs personal medical, health, dietary, exercise, or other assistance or advice, the reader should consult a competent physician and/or other qualified health care professionals. The author and publisher specifically disclaim all responsibility for injury, damage, or loss that the reader may incur as a direct or indirect consequence of following any directions or suggestions given in the book or participating in any programs described in the book.

ULTRA-PROCESSED FOODS: Concerns, Controversies, and Exceptions. Copyright © 2026 by NutritionFacts.org. All rights reserved. Printed in the United States of America. For information, address NutritionFacts.org, P.O. Box 11400, Takoma Park, MD 20913.

LCCN 2025925153
ISBN 979-8-9916605-2-5 (paperback)
ISBN 979-8-9916605-3-2 (e-book)
The Library of Congress Cataloging-in-Publication Data is available upon request.

First paperback edition, January 2026

Cover design, figures, and charts by Robert King Design. Cover art by Kat Farrell, NutritionFacts.org. Interior by Typeflow.

CONTENTS

INTRODUCTION

A century ago, modern nutrition science arose in the context of nutrient deficiency.[1] Editorials in the *Journal of the American Medical Association* had titles like "Sugar as Food," heralding sugar as one of the cheapest sources of calories. For 10 cents, you could buy 3,000 calories.[2]

Then, the Nutrient Deficiency era gave way to the Dietary Excess era.[3] No longer were we dying of deficiency diseases like scurvy as much as we were dying from nutrient *excess* diseases like obesity and heart disease. So, dietary guidance became more about avoiding too many calories and too much saturated fat, sugar, and sodium, though it maintained its focus on nutrients.[4] That allowed food manufacturers to get away with launching the likes of fat-free SnackWell's cookies. Food, however, not nutrients, can be considered the fundamental unit in nutrition,[5] and, to its credit, the field of nutrition started moving towards a more holistic view.[6]

First-generation dietary guidelines emphasized individual nutrients, like fat, then moved to second-generation *food*-based dietary guidance.[7] These largely converged on encouraging diets rich in fruits, vegetables, nuts, whole grains, and legumes—beans, split peas, chickpeas, and lentils. An area of emerging importance, however, is the degree of food processing.[8]

So, national nutrition guidelines started out telling us to cut down on sugar, salt, saturated fat, cholesterol, and alcohol, then moved to actually naming names, suggesting we might want to cut down on "cakes," for example. Guidance shifted from a focus on nutrients to foods. More recently, some countries have started recommending that we limit our intake of processed foods.[9]

Credited for starting the momentum was a commentary in the journal *Public Health Nutrition* in 2009 by Carlos Monteiro, a nutrition professor at the University of São Paulo in Brazil. He suggested the issue with nutrition and health was not so much the food, nor the nutrients, as much as the level of processing.[10]

To illustrate, a food-based dietary guideline might tell us to eat more vegetable soup.[11] Great! But there's vegetable soup, and then there's vegetable soup. Are we talking a clean-out-your-fridge vegetable soup? Or Amy's Organic health-haloed Quinoa, Kale & Red Lentil soup with a *heart-stopping* 1,240 milligrams of sodium per can?[12] Or Lipton vegetable soup that contains more salt than vegetables?[13] Or how about a vegetable-*flavored* soup that has more artificial flavors and MSG than veggies?[14] All soup is not the same. The level of processing matters. Similarly, there are breakfast cereals (single-ingredient shredded wheat), and then there are breakfast cereals (Marshmallow Fruity Pebbles).[15,16]

Professor Monteiro and colleagues proposed the *NOVA system of food classification*. Not an acronym, NOVA means *new* in Portuguese, as in a new way to classify foods, based on the level of processing. All foods and food products are classified into four groups, as shown in Figure 1.[17]

Group 1 foods are unprocessed or minimally processed. Think fresh, dried, frozen, or cooked plant or animal products, but nothing bad added, like salt or sugar. Group 2 foods are the salt, sugar, and fats used in cooking. Group 3 foods are traditionally processed ones, like when group 2 ingredients are added to group 1 foods. What really put NOVA on the map, however, is group 4, its concept of *ultra*-processed foods.[18]

Ultra-processed foods are industrial "formulations of several ingredients which, besides salt, sugar, oils and fats, include food substances not used in culinary preparations, in particular, flavours, colours, sweeteners, emulsifiers and other additives used to imitate" real foods.[19] Think Twinkies. Or a Frosted Wild Berry Pop-Tart that has more berries pictured on the front of its box than inside of it but may still taste like berries and look like berries because of no less than seven different artificial food dyes (and a natural color, carmine—made from red bugs).[20]

NOVA Classification System

Group 1

Unprocessed or Minimally Processed Foods

fresh, dry, or frozen vegetables or fruits; legumes; grains; nuts and seeds; meat (including fish); milk; eggs

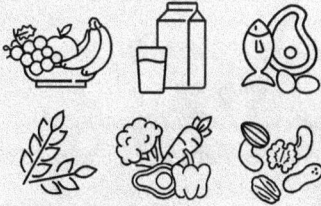

Processing includes the removal of inedible and other unwanted parts and does not add substances to the original food.

Group 2

Processed Culinary Ingredients

animal fats (e.g., butter, lard, cream), plant oils (e.g., olive oil, coconut oil), sugar, honey, maple syrup, and salt

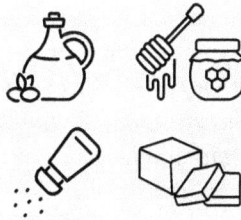

Group 2 products are substances derived from Group 1 foods or nature by processes such as refining, milling, pressing, grinding, and drying.

Group 3

Processed Foods

canned or pickled vegetables, fruits, or meat (including fish); cheese; salted meat; artisanal bread; beer, wine, and cider

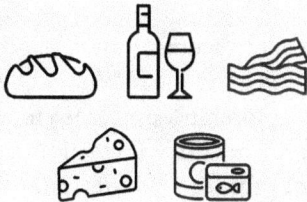

Group 3 products are processed from Group 1 or 2 foods with the addition of salt, oil, or sugar through canning, pickling, curing, fermenting, or smoking.

Group 4

Ultra-Processed Foods

sweet and savory snacks; ice cream; sugar-sweetened beverages; chicken nuggets; fish sticks; reconstituted meat products; instant or canned soups; prepared frozen foods

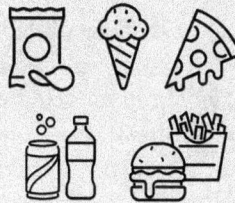

Group 4 products are made from a series of processes, including chemical modification and extraction, and contain very little intact Group 1 foods.

Figure 1

Ultra-processed foods can be so nutritionally vacuous that if they were all you ate, you could go blind from nutrient deficiencies. Sound like hyperbole? Tell that to the 17-year-old boy who apparently lived off french fries, Pringles, white bread, ham, and sausage and lost his vision.[21]

"Simply put," explained one public health journal commentary, "ultra-processed foods are foods that can't be made in your home kitchen because they have been chemically or physically transformed using industrial processes."[22] Monteiro and colleagues describe ultra-processed foods and beverages as:

> *"typically contain[ing] little or no whole foods, are ready-to-consume or heat up, and are fatty, salty or sugary and depleted in dietary fibre....Examples include: sweet, fatty or salty packaged snack products, ice cream, sugar-sweetened beverages, chocolates, confectionery, French fries, burgers and hot dogs, and poultry and fish nuggets."[23]*

Basically, nearly anything sold in a box or a bag. Why not just refer to them as "packaged foods"? That was considered, but public health advocates worried that consumers might look at a bag of apples and get confused.[24]

Before the NOVA classification system was introduced, the issue of food processing wasn't much on the radar.[25] But, when NOVA exploded onto the stage, it "resulted in a *superNOVA* in the world of nutrition."[26] Monteiro considers ultra-processed foods to have "troublesome" social, cultural, economic, political, and environmental implications.[27] In this book, however, I will focus on their health implications.

What exactly is so revolutionary about this concept of ultra-processed foods? Wasn't fatty, salty, sugary junk always a bad idea? What's so novel about NOVA? Monteiro claims that diets heavy in ultra-processed foods are *intrinsically* unhealthy and, in fact, there are harmful effects of ultra-processed foods "irrespective of their nutrient profiles."[28] Is this true?

THE ULTRA-PROCESSED PROBLEM

The United States has the lowest life expectancy of the top dozen most affluent countries in the world,[29] as well as a diet that contains the greatest share of ultra-processed foods. Most of what goes into American mouths isn't real food.[30] Could there be a connection between the two?

Based on studies encompassing nearly 10 million participants, higher consumption of ultra-processed foods is associated with a higher risk of a variety of disease outcomes, including all-cause mortality.[31] That means a greater intake of ultra-processed foods could be linked to living a significantly shorter life.

Some of the health problems make sense. Greater intake of ultra-processed foods is associated with more dental cavities in children, presumably thanks to the sugar,[32] and increased risk of high blood pressure, presumably thanks to the salt.[33] With higher blood pressure, it makes sense that there could be a higher rate of heart attacks and strokes. Since these are some of our leading killers, it also makes sense that excessive intake of ultra-processed foods could lead to increased overall mortality.[34]

Obesity is also a no-brainer. Not only are ultra-processed foods often packed with calories,[35] many are intentionally engineered with hyperpalatable, flavored, fatty, salty, sugary combinations so you crave more and more, thereby promoting weight gain through "hedonic eating"—eating for pleasure, even if you aren't really hungry.[36]

All that makes sense, but why would there also be a higher overall risk of cancer associated with ultra-processed food consumption?[37] Or a higher risk of dementia?[38] Or inflammatory bowel disease[39] or irritable bowel syndrome?[40] There's a higher risk of developing chronic kidney disease, too.[41] Overall, links have been found between the intake of ultra-processed foods and 71% of the health issues that have been investigated.

As shown in Figure 2, greater consumption of ultra-processed foods has been correlated with higher risks of dying from all causes put together; getting cancer; not sleeping well; suffering from anxiety, depression, and other common mental disorders; wheezing; cardiovascular disease; Crohn's disease; abdominal obesity and obesity in general; fatty liver disease; and type 2 diabetes.[42] There doesn't appear to be a single study linking ultra-processed food intake in general with any sort of beneficial health outcome.[43] There was never a *take two Twinkies and call me in the morning* kind of thing.

An international team of public health researchers concluded: "Given the large body of evidence implicating UPFs [ultra-processed foods] in human diseases, and the ever-increasing consumption of UPFs around the world, there is a pressing need to recognize the contribution of UPFs to the global burden of disease."[44] But wait. These are just *associations*.

Simply because A is correlated with B doesn't mean that A *causes* B. Maybe B causes A. For example, snapshot-in-time studies have shown that higher consumption of ultra-processed foods is associated with higher odds of depression and anxiety symptoms, but which came first? Who hasn't on occasion turned to fatty, sugary, salty junk when feeling stressed or anxious?[45] It's called *comfort food* for a reason.

There are longitudinal studies that have shown that greater consumption of ultra-processed foods *preceded* the depression, but perhaps the junky food had been used to fend off bad feelings for years before any official diagnosis.[46] Nevertheless, reverse causation—B causing A—seems less plausible when it comes to *non*-mental health outcomes. For example, it's harder to paint a picture of how a heart attack would cause people to then go on to eat more junk food instead of vice versa.

Confounding is another concern when trying to establish cause and effect from observational, correlational data. Perhaps the only reason A is associated with B is because a third confounding factor, C, is linked to both.

Significant Associations Between Greater Ultra-Processed Food Consumption and Adverse Health Outcomes

OUTCOME	EQUIVALENT ODDS RATIO (95% CI)
Mortality	
All-cause mortality	
Cardiovascular disease-related mortality	
Heart disease-related mortality	
Cancer	
Cancer (overall)	
Colorectal cancer	
Cardiovascular Health	
Cardiovascular disease events combined	
Cardiovascular disease morbidity	
Hypertension	
Low HDL cholesterol	
Gastrointestinal Health	
Crohn's disease	
Mental Health	
Adverse sleep-related outcomes	
Anxiety outcomes	
Common mental disorder outcomes	
Depressive outcomes	
Metabolic Health	
Abdominal obesity	
Metabolic syndrome	
Non-alcoholic fatty liver disease	
Obesity	
Overweight	
Overweight + obesity	
Type 2 diabetes	
Respiratory Health	
Wheezing	

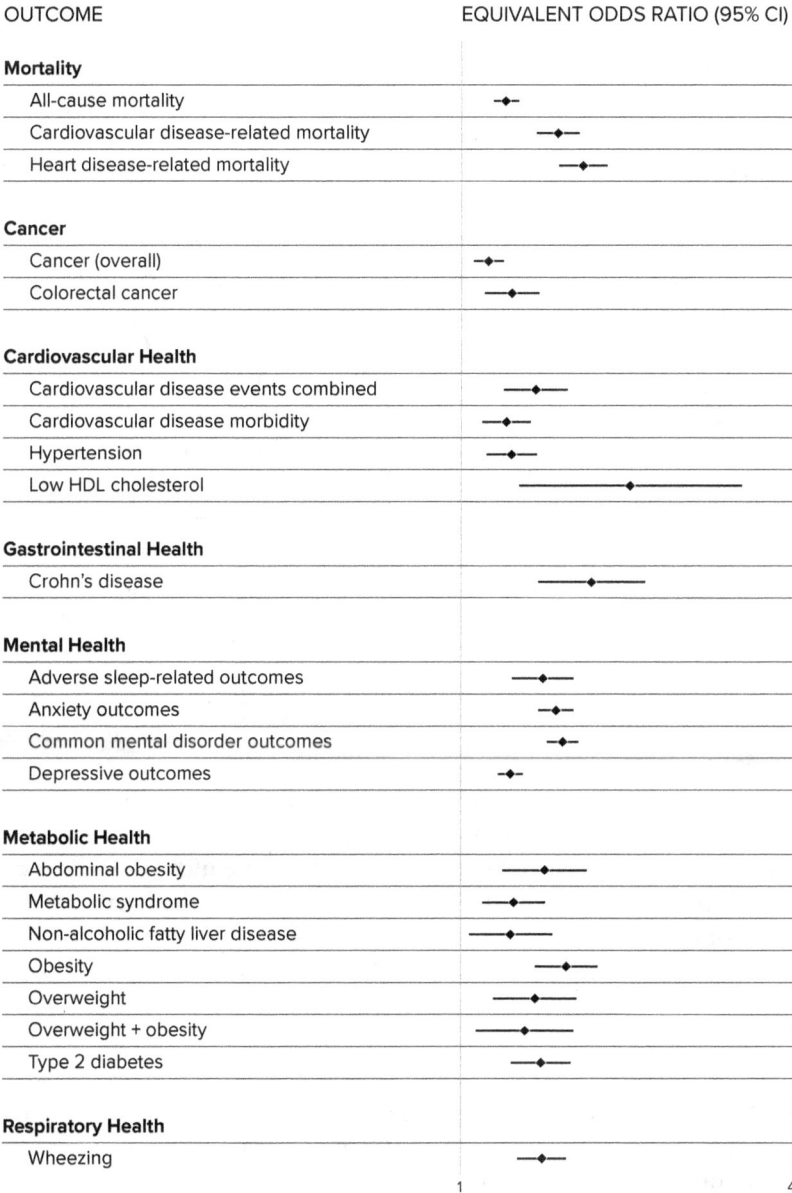

1   4

Figure 2

For example, if people who eat more junk tend to smoke more, it's unsurprising that they would be dying more, but the deaths might have more to do with the cigarettes they put in their mouth rather than the food.

People with unhealthy diets are more likely to smoke, drink, and not exercise,[47,48] but we have ways to control for these factors.[49] Indeed, the majority of studies on ultra-processed foods and disease outcomes were adjusted for these confounders. The most obvious one, though, is that highly processed foods are more likely to be junky.

Might the reason cakes, crullers, candy, and cola are bad for us have less to do with how much they've been processed and more to do with the fact they are *cakes, crullers, candy, and cola*—packed with sugar and calories, with very few nutrients?[50] Diets high in ultra-processed foods are diets high in added sugars, saturated fat, sodium, and empty calories that displace more healthful foods like fruits and vegetables, so maybe ultra-processed foods are merely markers of poor diets.[51] The more ultra-processed foods we eat, the more added sugar we tend to get in our diets, the more sodium, saturated fat, cholesterol, and refined carbohydrates, and the less fiber.[52] So where is the mystery? People who eat lots of unhealthy foods tend to become unhealthy. We already knew that. What does processing have to do with it?

Foods in the ultra-processed category are more likely to be junky, so we could use it as a kind of heuristic that they probably aren't good for us.[53] If you made a rule to avoid breakfast cereals with cartoon character mascots, you'd probably be healthier, but not because the graven image of Tony the Tiger is hastening you to the grave, but rather because it's a proxy for high sugar content. However, for the developers of the ultra-processed concept, *ultra-processed* was no proxy. They claimed that the harmful effects of ultra-processed foods are not fully captured by their nutrient labels and went so far as to say we should minimize our intake, "irrespective of their nutrient profiles."[54]

Are ultra-processed foods bad for us just because their nutritional quality is poor, or does processing itself have health consequences? How might we settle this? Well, if it were the case that the association between ultra-processed foods and poor health was solely due to a generally less healthful diet, then that association should disappear if we were to adjust for dietary quality. In other words, if it were all about nutrients, then people eating crappy diets high in sugar, salt, and saturated fat should have high disease rates regardless of their intake of ultra-processed foods, and people who eat really healthful diets should have low rates of disease regardless of how many ultra-processed foods they consume, but that doesn't appear to be the case.[55]

A review of the evidence found that the majority of the links between ultra-processed foods and health problems "remain significant and unchanged in magnitude after adjustment for diet quality or pattern," meaning that even if we balance out dietary quality, those eating more ultra-processed foods do tend to fare worse. This suggests that at least some of the adverse consequences of ultra-processed foods are independent of dietary quality, so ultra-processed food companies can't simply reformulate their products to be lower in salt or sugar and be done with it.[56] There appears to be something about this class of foods beyond the standard nutrient profile that contributes to their deleterious effects.

POTENTIAL DRIVERS OF DISEASE

Ultra-processed foods may not be "real food," but they can really affect our health. Why do we need a new term, though? Isn't it enough to just say we should stay away from junk food?

Junk is defined as foods and beverages with high levels of concentrated calories and added saturated fats, sodium, and sugar. It's the source of most of Americans' sugar and about half of our calories, salt, and saturated fat.[57] But *ultra-processed* is not synonymous with *junk*. Some junk foods are not ultra-processed, and some ultra-processed foods don't fit the definition of junk.

For example, while sausage is considered an ultra-processed meat, bacon is considered just a processed meat, though bacon would also meet junk food's definition of a calorie-concentrated food loaded with added salt.[58] Conversely, consider an ultra-processed product like Diet Coke. It doesn't have any calories, sugar, or fat. Therefore, it's not technically junk, but it's still not necessarily harmless. So, there's a limitation to exclusively focusing on the nutrient profile of ultra-processed foods,[59] but how can an ultra-processed product be bad if it's fat-free, sugar-free, and salt-free?

Food Additives

The health risks of ultra-processed foods are not only related to their poor nutritional quality, but also to the presence of additives.[60] Diet Coke may not have any apparent calories, fat, sugar, or salt, but it does contain caramel color,[61] which results in the formation of 4-methylimidazole,[62] a possible human carcinogen.[63] It contains aspartame, too,[64] which has also been classified as possibly cancer-causing in humans.[65]

Diet Coke also contains phosphoric acid,[66] a harmful phosphate additive[67] that could help explain the link between ultra-processed foods intake and problems with our heart and kidneys.[68]

Diet Coke also contains a benzoate preservative.[69] When researchers removed artificial colorings and benzoate preservatives from preschoolers' diets and then randomized the kids to be given a placebo or a cocktail of colorings and benzoate, one measure of hyperactivity was reduced significantly while the children were on the removal diet free of colorings and benzoates yet increased significantly when the additives were added back in, compared to placebo.[70] Of course, it could have been the colorings, not the benzoate, but that's one of the problems. As little as we know about the effects of these individual additives, we know even less about what combinations of them can do.[71]

There is a large body of evidence that suggests toxicity from certain artificial food colorings, benzoate preservatives, and artificial sweeteners, sometimes through adverse effects on our gut microbiome.[72] This may explain at least some of the apparent connection between inflammatory bowel disease and ultra-processed foods intake.[73]

Industry apologists argue that the U.S. Food and Drug Administration (FDA) "carefully evaluates" food additives to make sure they are safe. To show the system works, they cite the removal in 2018 of six artificial flavors found to be carcinogenic.[74] However, those additives were approved for safety and in the food supply beginning in 1964,[75] so we were exposed to them for more than 50 years before they were banned. And that's their example of the system working!

Critics of the ultra-processed foods concept question why yogurt with artificial sweetener is smeared with the ultra-processed label when it contains less sugar than regular yogurt.[76] You can see how they are trying to stick with the nutrient paradigm of *less sugar should be better.* But that was before aspartame, widely sold as NutraSweet, was officially recognized as a potential human carcinogen in 2023.[77]

Forty-two years earlier, when aspartame was first approved, the FDA's own public board of inquiry opposed its approval based on brain tumors in rats in the industry's own studies. The FDA Commissioner summarily rejected these concerns and approved the sweetener anyway before leaving the agency for a $1,000 per day consultancy position with the aspartame company's public relations firm. The FDA then prevented the National Toxicology Program from conducting further cancer testing.[78] Meanwhile, tens of millions of pounds of aspartame made its way into the food supply each year.[79]

Critics of the ultra-processed label argue that, if some additives are bad, we just need to identify them and get rid of them.[80] Instead of the *guilty until proven innocent* approach, we should not broad-brush all additives as potentially harmful. But what about artificial food colors? What level of evidence do we need to remove something that exists to make rainbow marshmallows in kids' cereals that much more eye-catching?

I've long been concerned that Red Dye No. 3 can still be in our food,[81] given that it was banned more than 30 years ago from inclusion in anything going on our skin due to cancer risk. It is considered too dangerous to apply topically, but it's okay to eat? Finally, in 2025, the FDA agreed to ban it from food, 35 years after banning it from cosmetics.[82] The ban goes into effect in 2027. Until then, here's a suggestion for food companies: Want to make your cherry popsicles red? Try adding some cherries.

If the harm of ultra-processed foods lies in potentially harmful additives, why not just stick to "clean label foods," made with simple and recognizable ingredients, no matter how the food is processed?[83] That assumes additives are the only reason ultra-processed foods may be unhealthy. In fact, harmful additives are just one of many reasons ultra-processed foods may lead to increased risk of death and disease.[84]

Processing Contaminants

At least food additives are listed in the ingredients on product labels so we can avoid them if we so choose. Unlisted are some of the sneakier ways ultra-processed foods may harm us. For instance, contaminants that are formed during industrial processing methods.[85]

Acrolein, for example, is a toxin found in cigarette smoke. It's also generated when frying or cooking with oils or other fats.[86] So, acrolein can be found in such foods as french fries, donuts, and potato chips.[87] This toxin appears to contribute to cancer[88] and cardiovascular disease risk.[89] (Ironically, canola oil, considered to be perhaps the most heart-healthy oil,[90] appears to generate among the highest amounts of acrolein.[91]) In fairness, acrolein formation would still be a problem if you made french fries from scratch, which would be considered a minimally processed food.[92] But if we had to cut up potatoes and deep fry them ourselves every time we wanted some, we'd probably eat a lot fewer of them.

Fried and pre-fried foods may also be contaminated with 3-MCPD, another possible carcinogen.[93] Furans and acrylamide are two other heat-generated contaminants[94] that are possibly or probably cancer-causing.[95,96]

Many readers will be aware of the fact that added trans fats were banned in 2021.[97] Unfortunately, trans fats are still produced[98] in the refining process of making vegetable oils,[99] so they may end up being as much as 0.5% trans fats. That said, even unprocessed meat and dairy can naturally contain 10 times more trans fats,[100] so they are now the major dietary source in the United States.[101]

Animal products—meat, eggs, and dairy—can also contain cholesterol oxidation products, which have been found to play a role in the progression of several inflammatory diseases.[102] *Oxidized* cholesterol appears to be even more pathogenic than regular cholesterol.[103] It's associated with both the initiation and progression of such major chronic diseases as Alzheimer's, atherosclerosis, diabetes, and kidney failure.[104]

Food processing can dramatically trigger the accumulation of cholesterol oxidation products in meats, including fish and poultry, eggs, and dairy products—even if the "processing" is just cooking,[105] with maximal cholesterol oxidation at only around 300°F (150°C).[106] Hence, the difference between their levels in an ultra-processed product like pork sausage isn't that different from a minimally processed product like roast pork.[107] So, many of these contaminants are not exclusive to ultra-processed foods. That's also the case with advanced glycation end-products (AGEs).[108]

There is growing evidence that intake of dietary AGEs is related closely to the occurrence of such chronic diseases as osteoporosis, diabetes, Alzheimer's, and chronic kidney disease.[109] A research perspective in a geriatric medicine journal suggested: "It is hard to find an age-related disease that AGEs are not involved...."[110] So, how can we avoid them?

Dietary AGEs are found in abundance in highly processed foods.[111] The food industry commonly uses "thermal treatments" to improve flavor and texture, as well as preservation and food safety—but *thermal treatment* just means heat. So, AGEs can arise from both industrial processing and home cooking.[112] As important as the level of processing, or even more so, may be the source—plant versus animal.

Canned corn, for example, has 20 units of AGEs per serving, corn chips 151, and corn pops cereal 373. Rice has 9 AGE units per serving, rice crackers have 275, and Rice Krispies 600. A boiled potato has 17 units per serving, potato chips 865, and fast-food fries more than 1,500. So, ultra-processed plant foods can have nearly a hundred times more AGE units than minimally processed plant foods, but animal foods start out with high levels even when they're raw and unprocessed, and just go up from there.[113]

Instead of the 9 AGE units of cooked rice or the 20 units of cooked corn, raw fish, poultry, and other meats start out with AGE units around 500 or more; once cooked, AGE levels jump into the thousands, yet those foods are still considered minimally processed. For meat that is processed or ultra-processed, the level can exceed 10,000 AGE units per serving.[114]

Although these contaminants are by no means limited to ultra-processed foods,[115] one can see how only considering nutrition labels and ingredient lists fails to capture how food processing "transforms food at the molecular level."[116] The clean label strategy of sticking to foods with simple ingredient lists won't help because we're not going to see acrolein or acrylamide listed on labels.[117] It's the processing itself, whether traditional or industrial, that is affecting the healthfulness of the food.

Packaging Chemicals

The contaminants that migrate into food from packaging materials are also not included on product labels. These include bisphenols like BPA, microplastics and plastics compounds like phthalates, as well as mineral oils.[118]

Evidently, the mineral oils can come from printing inks from the recycled newspapers used in paperboard packaging, which can then migrate into the food.[119] They accumulate in our own tissues to levels that have been found to be harmful in a certain strain of rats.[120] (The relevance to humans has been questioned since the results can't even be extrapolated from one strain of rats to another.[121])

Plastic packaging can contain thousands of different molecules, of which more than 300 are already considered as potentially risky to our health.[122] These include phthalates, which, along with bisphenols, may have hormone-modulating effects.[123] It doesn't take long to clear them from our system, though. When study participants switched from packaged foods to fresh foods, evidence of their exposure to phthalate and bisphenol, based on urine samples, dropped significantly within just a few days.[124]

Although phthalates are best known as hormone disrupters, with potential testicular toxicity, ovarian toxicity, and endometriosis risk, there's also a concern about kidney toxicity, nerve damage, liver damage, and heart damage.[125] Exposure to BPA, the best-studied bisphenol, is associated with congenital abnormalities, diabetes, polycystic ovary syndrome, obesity, and cardiovascular disease.[126]

At first, scientists didn't think the migration of BPA into foods was sufficient to exceed safety levels, but newer data have raised some alarm bells. We not only now have evidence of potential harm from levels of BPA in foods that are well below current regulations, but also well below levels to which we as consumers have been regularly exposed.[127] Yet, we continue to produce millions of tons of it each year,[128] so it's no surprise that about 90% of Americans have at least trace levels of BPAs flowing through us at any given time,[129] depending in part on what we eat. BPA is often used to line cans, so researchers randomized study participants to eat a serving of canned soup every day for five days and saw a 1,000% rise in their BPA levels, compared to those eating soups made with fresh ingredients.[130]

Looking at the associations between the consumption of ultra-processed foods and how many phthalates and bisphenols are flowing through our system, researchers found higher levels of four phthalates and the bisphenol BPF associated with higher intake of ultra-processed foods. However, they found a lack of association with the most common ones, DEHP and BPA, as well as an inverse association for the bisphenol BPS, meaning the more ultra-processed one's diet, the lower the exposure.[131] This makes sense since, in the food supply, BPS has only been found in meat, most of which is considered minimally processed.[132] Similarly, DEHP levels are associated with consuming poultry, where some of the highest levels of DEHP per serving are found.[133] That helps explain why eating vegetarian for a few days can lead to significant decreases in phthalate exposure.[134] The lack of correlation between BPA and ultra-processed food intake may be because only about half of canned foods tested for BPA were ultra-processed.[135]

We can look for *BPA-free* on the labels of canned goods, just as we can scan the ingredients list for additives we now know may be harmful. But do you see the problem? Many contaminants and additives were considered harmless, until they weren't, like BPA, aspartame, and the artificial colors and flavors that flooded the food supply for decades before they were banned.

Remember when the food industry thought partially hydrogenating vegetable oils were a good idea and replaced the saturated fat in tropical oils with trans fats from partially hydrogenated oils? Although many countries now restrict the use of trans fats, they continue to kill an estimated half a million people around the world each year.[136] Of course, excess saturated fat probably also kills hundreds of thousands a year,[137] but the point is that trans fats from partially hydrogenated vegetable oil killed people for decades before any limits were placed on them. The FDA didn't ban trans fats until more than 25 years *after* the first solid evidence emerged that it increased the risk of heart disease. From the time we knew until the time it was banned, trans fats were killing up to 50,000 Americans annually.[138] That's quite the death toll that can be laid at the feet of the ultra-processed food industry.

The retort from industry was *but we originally thought trans fats were safe!* That's the problem. Anytime some chemical company develops a new preservative or sweetener or artificial color, we have no idea how it will eventually turn out decades later. So, you can start to see the value of this ultra-processed food concept where an entire category of products is essentially presumed guilty until proven innocent. That drives the food industry crazy but look at its track record. Look at the trail of bodies it's left behind.

Loss of Phytonutrients

There is an outdated view of nutrition and public health that we just have to tick off all the basic nutrient boxes for health and wellness.[139] This notion allows food manufacturers like General Mills to boast that its Lucky Charms' marshmallows aren't only "brighter" but fortified with 12 essential vitamins and minerals.[140] Those with ties to candy bar companies[141] argue that ultra-processed foods have essential nutrients, but essential nutrients are just the tip of the iceberg when it comes to the number and variety of compounds in whole foods.[142]

Ultra-processed foods don't only negatively impact nutritional status through a relative lack of micronutrients, like essential vitamins and minerals; they also lack phytonutrients, the thousands of plant nutrients that aren't listed on the ingredients label but may benefit our health.[143] For instance, polyphenols. They aren't technically essential in that they are not necessary for life, but they may be necessary for long life, so they may be considered "lifespan essentials."[144]

Only about 150 nutritional components of foods are commonly measured and tracked, yet they represent a tiny fraction of the more than 26,000 compounds present in our food—many with documented health effects.[145] There are more than 8,000 kinds of polyphenols alone.[146] Flavonoids are part of this "dark matter of nutrition."[147] They're a subset of polyphenols found in fruits, vegetables, whole grains, herbs, and teas that may help explain why these foods and beverages may have protective effects against some of our leading killers, like cancer and Alzheimer's. Unsurprisingly, those who consume the most ultra-processed products get significantly fewer flavonoids in their diet.[148]

Consider garlic. Nutrient databases may tell us that it has manganese, vitamin B6, and selenium, but a clove of garlic contains more than 2,000 distinct components[149] that are presumably responsible for the cancer protection associated with eating garlic family vegetables and the beneficial cardiometabolic effects seen when garlic was actually put to the test in clinical trials.[150] But when the amount of garlic extract in a food is less than the amount of MSG (as may be typical in a bag of flavored potato chips), we're probably going to miss out on its benefits.[151]

Here's a life and death example. When brown rice started to be polished into white rice, people started dying en masse from a nutrient deficiency disease called beriberi.[152] It became one of the most common diseases in Asia. During the milling process, the rice germ and bran are removed and, with them, the B vitamin thiamin.[153] Today, white rice is "enriched" by adding back the thiamin that had been stolen, but what about all the other phytonutrients that were removed?[154] And that's just going from brown rice to white, which is considered a moderate level of processing. Think how much is lost when rice is turned into an ultra-processed product like brown rice syrup or when a whole soybean is processed into something like soy lecithin.

Just as our bodies are not used to all the new stuff *added* to our foods, our bodies aren't used to having all the original components like fiber *subtracted* from what we eat. Just as it's difficult to tease out the long-term consequences of the cocktails of new food additives, we don't know what critical combinations of phytonutrients we may be missing in these new ultra-processed products.[155] Until Big Food figures it out and can add a lucky 13th marshmallow mineral or vitamin, it may be best to try to prioritize whole foods.

Changes in Texture

One of the mechanisms linking increased consumption of ultra-processed foods and increased risk of death and disease is calorie overload, which leads to excess body fat.[156] To date, all prospective population studies on ultra-processed food consumption and weight gain have found that the more ultra-processed foods we eat, the more likely we are to become overweight or obese.[157] One reason we tend to overconsume ultra-processed foods more than less-processed foods may be their texture.[158]

When study participants were served a dish made with soft, creamy risotto rice and boiled vegetables, they ate 17% more calories than when they were given the same dish made with regular rice and raw vegetables. They even ate more when just their hamburger bun was soft, compared to hard.[159] What does Big Food tend to dish out for us? Products processed for maximum consumption rate. It's called *fast food* for a reason. Unlike foods made in factories, foods that *grow* tend to be slow. Thanks in part to the fiber content of whole, healthy plant foods, the default eating rate of more healthful foods tends to be slower, naturally.[160]

Though there are certainly exceptions, like caramel toffee, highly processed foods tend to be consumed quickly. There can be a hundredfold difference in consumption between the fastest and slowest foods. In just four minutes, you could consume 2,000 calories of chocolate milk, an entire day's worth of calories, but it could take about *eight hours* to eat 2,000 calories of raw carrots.[161,162,163]

Based on an analysis of hundreds of different foods, the average caloric intake rate of ultra-processed foods is about double that of unprocessed foods, 69 versus 36 calories per minute, respectively.[164] Might that have less to do with the eating rate and more to do with how concentrated in calories so many ultra-processed foods are? They are often packed with added sugar and fat, not to mention salt and flavor enhancers, to help trigger compulsive eating. How might we tease out all these factors?

In a landmark study, people were assigned, in random order, a diet composed of either ultra-processed foods or unprocessed foods for two weeks, but the two diets were matched for presented calories, carbohydrates, protein, fat, sugar, salt, and fiber. So, if people overeat ultra-processed foods because of their junky nutrient profile and not their degree of processing, then the unprocessed foods diet matched in calories and nutrients would be expected to have similar results. But that wasn't the case. The study participants ate an average of 500 more calories each day on the ultra-processed diet and started gaining about a pound a week, while those on the unprocessed diet lost about a pound a week. So, within two weeks, there was already a four-pound difference between the two groups.[165]

Given that the two menus were matched for sugar, fat, and salt, why did people overeat the ultra-processed foods? It isn't because the ultra-processed foods were significantly more delicious; the diets were successfully matched for palatability, too. What differed was eating rate. People consumed calories 50% faster on the ultra-processed diet compared to the unprocessed diet.[166] And we know that the faster we eat, the more calories we tend to take in, presumed to be because our natural satiety mechanisms don't have time to catch up.[167] There are two other reasons that help explain why study participants gained so much more weight eating the ultra-processed diet: increased calorie density and the degradation of the food matrix, which I'll explain below.

High Calorie Density

Calorie density is the number of calories for a given weight or volume of food. As you can see in Figure 3, some foods have more calories per cup, per pound, per mouthful than others.

Oil, for example, has a high calorie density. That means a lot of calories are concentrated into a small space. Drizzling just one tablespoon of oil on a dish, for example, adds 120 calories.[168] For those same 120 calories, you could eat about *two cups* of blackberries, a food with a low calorie

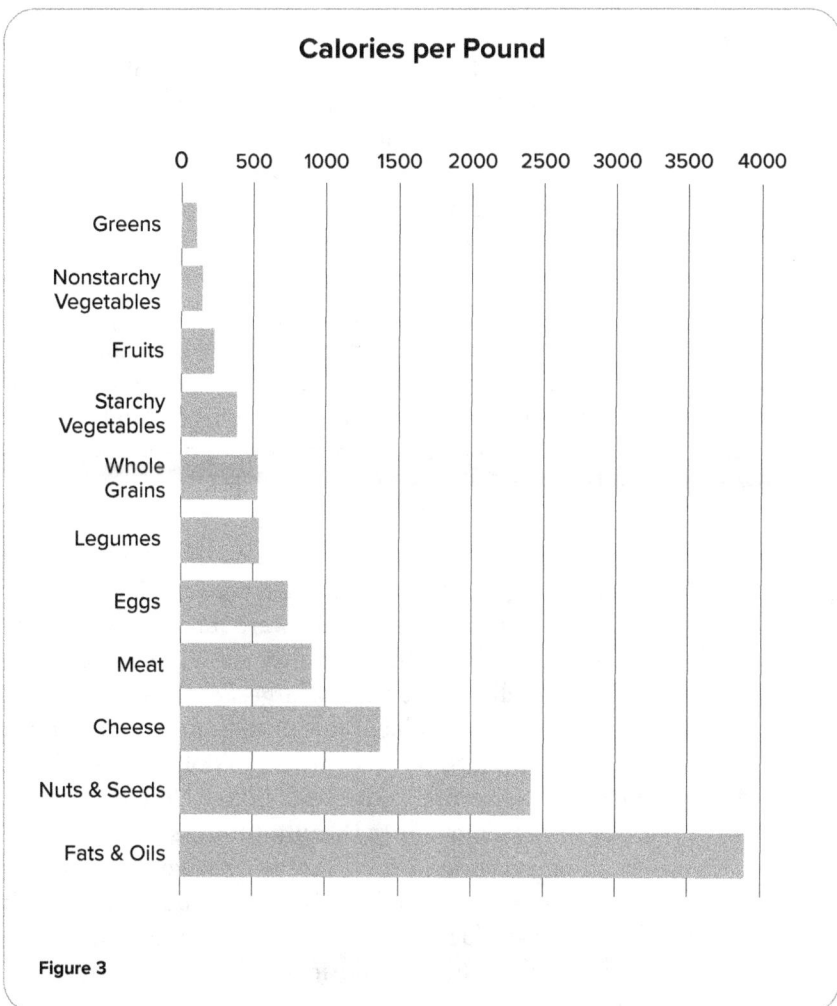

Calories per Pound

Greens	
Nonstarchy Vegetables	
Fruits	
Starchy Vegetables	
Whole Grains	
Legumes	
Eggs	
Meat	
Cheese	
Nuts & Seeds	
Fats & Oils	

Figure 3

density.[169] You could swig down that spoonful of oil and not even feel a difference, but eating a couple cups of berries could start to fill you up.

A handful of jelly beans has about 16 times more calories than a handful of cherry tomatoes.[170,171] For the same number of calories, you could eat that one handful of jelly beans or about four cups of cherry tomatoes. A large serving of french fries is about the same size and weight as a baked potato, but it has about four times the calories.[172,173] So, for the same number of calories, you could have that single serving of fries or around four baked potatoes. Which do you think would be more filling?

Ultra-processed foods tend to have twice the calorie density compared to unprocessed foods, more than 1,000 calories per pound.[174] That's similar to what you see at fast-food joints, whereas traditional rural West African diets, which closely represent the likely diet of our ancient ancestors, average fewer than 500 calories per pound.[175]

The biological mechanisms our bodies use to regulate our weight likely evolved in the context of eating at least four or five pounds of food a day.[176] That may be the amount of food that's more natural for us to consume. If our body is counting on eating five pounds of food, but we max out with the same number of calories eating just two pounds of ultra-processed food,[177] what do you think happens? It's no wonder we overeat—our bodies are expecting three more pounds of food! We just weren't designed to handle such calorie-concentrated diets. No wonder ultra-processed foods are so fattening.

But what about the study I just discussed, where people ended up four pounds heavier within two weeks eating an ultra-processed diet compared to an unprocessed diet, even though the menus were supposedly matched for calorie density? A typical meal in the ultra-processed group included a deli meat and cheese quesadilla compared to a large, Southwestern entrée salad with black beans, nuts, avocados, corn, grapes, and apples in the unprocessed group. How could those two meals possibly be matched in calorie density, the same number of calories per pound? The researchers added five cups of sugar-free lemonade to the ultra-processed meal to help even out the calories per total poundage.[178] That seems like cheating. Calorie density shouldn't be based on food *and* beverages, but, ideally, only on food because beverages are so heavy just from their water content that they can disproportionately influence calorie density calculations. If we look only at the calorie density of the food in the study,[179] the *non-beverage* calorie density was 85% higher on the ultra-processed foods diet, which could account for some of that weight gain.[180]

You can't fault the researchers for trying the diet lemonade trick. High calorie density is such an inherent property of so many ultra-processed foods. How else could you actually match them with a variety of unprocessed foods? And that's the problem. High calorie density is one of the reasons ultra-processed foods may be contributing to the obesity epidemic.[181]

Changes in Structure

The landmark study that found that ultra-processed foods caused excess weight gain compared to unprocessed foods matched the menus for the amounts of calories, sugar, fat, and fiber on offer. How exactly did the researchers match for fiber content?[182] It's hard to imagine ultra-processed foods having much fiber, which is naturally concentrated in only one place: whole plant foods.

Rounding out a representative ultra-processed dinner with a deli meat and cheese sandwich and cups of diet lemonade was nonfat yogurt, fruit in heavy syrup, and baked potato chips. How could the ultra-processed meal possibly have the same amount of fiber as the unprocessed meal with the Southwestern entrée salad with beans, greens, nuts, fruits, and vegetables? The researchers added a fiber supplement powder to the yogurt and lemonade.[183] So, technically, both meals had the same amount of fiber.

But that's not how fiber works.

A half century ago, the *dietary fiber hypothesis* was proposed,[184] suggesting that fiber is the reason that diets centered around whole plant foods are so protective against chronic disease.[185] Predictably, this gave rise to a multibillion-dollar fiber supplement market.[186] We could just eat real food, but when there's money to be made, there are supplements to be sold.

Those who get more fiber in their diet do appear to be significantly less likely to suffer from heart disease, strokes, and diabetes. They are also less likely to die from cancer and all causes put together. But the studies that find these protective effects for fiber were all looking at fiber intake from food. For both disease prevention and treatment, evidence suggests fiber supplements are no substitute.[187] To understand why you can't just chase your slice of Wonder Bread with some Metamucil, one has to understand how fiber works.

Dietary fiber alone has certain benefits, but its primary role may be to physically encapsulate nutrients inside cell walls for special delivery to our gut microbiome. The cells of plants are encased in walls made out of fiber, which act as an indigestible physical barrier, so when we eat structurally intact plant foods, many of the nutrients remain trapped. We can chew all we want, but we'll still end up with nutrients completely surrounded by fiber, which then blunts the glycemic response, activates a natural satiety mechanism called the *ileal brake*, and delivers sustenance to our friendly flora.[188] Like nature intended.

This may be why apples are more satiating than apple juice even when the juice is enriched with an identical amount of added fiber.[189] Structure matters. You can't just sprinkle on the fiber—it's part of the matrix. The word *matrix* comes from the Latin *matricis,* derived from *mater,* meaning "mother."[190] We should strive to preserve the matrix (the *blue* pill, Neo) by choosing more unprocessed plant foods.

Even with identical chemistry, food structure may result in major differences in health outcomes.[191] Corn chips and corn flakes cause a higher blood sugar spike (i.e., have a higher *glycemic index*) compared to corn on the cob. In fact, even with identical ingredients, food structure can make a difference.[192] Rolled oats, for example, have a significantly lower glycemic index than unsweetened instant oatmeal, which is also just straight oats but in thinner flakes.[193] Likewise, oat flakes have a lower glycemic index than oat powder.[194] The same single ingredient, oats, but in different forms can have different effects.

Why do we care? Because the hormonal and metabolic changes triggered by the overly rapid absorption of carbohydrates promote overeating. In a study out of Harvard's Children's Hospital, a dozen obese teen boys were fed instant oatmeal or steel-cut oatmeal. After the instant oatmeal, the teens went on to eat 53% more over the subsequent five hours than after eating the steel-cut oatmeal. The instant oatmeal group started snacking within an hour after their meal and ultimately accumulated significantly more calories throughout the rest of the day.[195]

Steel-cut oatmeal is considered a low-glycemic-index food, averaging under 55, whereas instant oatmeal is a high-glycemic food, averaging over 70. Some cold cereals can be worse, even zero-sugar cereals like shredded wheat.[196] The new industrial methods used to create breakfast cereals, such as extrusion cooking and explosion puffing, accelerate starch digestion and absorption, causing an exaggerated blood sugar response.[197] Shredded wheat has the same ingredients as spaghetti—straight wheat—but a 70% higher glycemic index.[198] This is one of the reasons processing matters. Food *structure* can play an important role in optimal health.[199]

Eating whole grains is good, but eating whole-grain *kernels* is better. Former chair of Harvard's nutrition department Walter Willett has argued that the term *whole grain* should probably be reserved for whole, intact grain kernels.[200] So, we should eat the wholiest of grains: intact grains, also known as *groats*.

A breakfast including whole rye kernels was found to result in increased feelings of satiety in the afternoon, compared to a morning meal of porridge made of whole-grain rye flour.[201] Instead of buying boxed breakfast cereals, make oatmeal out of whole, intact oats. *They're gr-r-oat!*

Addictive Properties

Another factor that may link increased consumption of ultra-processed foods with health harms is compulsive eating.[202]

It matters whether or not ultra-processed foods are considered addictive. Identifying tobacco products as not only unhealthy but addictive undermined the industry's claim that smoking was solely an act of free choice.[203] It's interesting: The food industry didn't just use the tobacco industry's playbook in marketing ultra-processed foods, like disproportionately targeting communities of color.[204] It *was* the tobacco industry.[205]

The rise in ultra-processed foods coincides with major tobacco corporations acquiring large food companies and becoming the biggest producers of ultra-processed foods.[206] Phillip Morris bought major U.S. food companies, including Kraft and General Foods, making the tobacco giant the largest food company in the world. RJ Reynolds, the largest tobacco company in the United States, purchased Nabisco and doubled company food profits in a single year.[207]

Product formulation strategies were learned from company scientists, included adding a variety of appealing colors to sugar-sweetened beverages.[208] Many of today's leading children's drink brands—Hawaiian Punch, Kool-Aid, and Capri Sun—were developed by tobacco companies.[209] They added caffeine and extra sugar to products to maximize consumption,[210] just as the tobacco industry manipulated nicotine levels in cigarettes to keep users smoking and convert as many as possible into heavy users.[211]

Not all foods have addictive potential. People don't tend to compulsively crave cabbage or binge on bananas. Highly processed foods appear to be most linked to addictive-like eating attributes, such as loss of control, though some less-processed, salty, fatty foods like cheese and bacon also fit the bill.[212] A study funded by the National Institute of Drug Abuse titled "Which Foods May Be Addictive?" ranked dozens of foods based on reports of problematic, addictive-type behaviors from hundreds of individuals and found that 100% of the top 10 most problematic foods were ultra-processed, whereas 100% of the 10 least problematic foods were not.[213]

How exactly are ultra-processed foods formulated to be "addictively" delicious, so you can't eat just one?[214] They're intentionally created to be hyperpalatable through the addition of fats, sugar, salt, and refined carbohydrates like white flour.[215] The combination of refined carbs and fats seems to have a particular effect on the reward systems in our brain, which may increase the addictive potential of these foods.[216] Few may sit down to enjoy a bowl of straight sugar or a tub of shortening, but put them together and you get frosting!

Why don't we crave trail mix as much? That's about as sugary and fatty as natural foods get. The key appears to lie in the processing, which increases the dose and speed of absorption of that sugar and fat. Hard liquor is more addictive than beer because of the dose, and crack is more addictive than cocaine because of the speed of absorption. Food processing can increase both of those simultaneously, delivering high loads of concentrated sugar and fat, while, at the same time, stripping away fiber, protein, and water to maximize the rate of absorption.[217]

There was an exponential increase in scientific publications on food addiction following the 2007 publication[218] of the pivotal study entitled "Intense Sweetness Surpasses Cocaine Reward,"[219] which found that when rats were allowed to choose between sweetened water or intravenous cocaine, 9 out of 10 chose the sweet taste over one of our most addictive drugs. People have been chewing coca leaves for a thousand years[220] as a mild stimulant without any evidence of addiction,[221] but when certain components in the plant were processed into a concentrated form for rapid delivery, the story took a harrowing turn.[222]

As with many drugs of abuse, salt, sugar, and fat are substances found in nature, but they exist naturally in much smaller concentrations and may only become problematic when extracted and concentrated by modern industrial processes.[223] Sugarcane stem has been chewed for its pleasant taste for ages,[224] but it only presents a disproportionate reward signal once it's been highly refined into added sugars with the potential to override our self-control mechanisms and, thus, lead to analogous addictive-type behaviors.[225] There's a reason we're more likely to supersize soda than sweet potatoes.

It was healthy and adaptive for our primate brains to search out sweetness in the form of a banana, but now that fruit is in Loop form, "this adaptation has become a dangerous liability," concluded National Institute on Drug Abuse researchers.[226]

Are Ultra-Processed Foods Addictive?

Food tastes good for the same reason sex feels good. We wouldn't last very long as a species without both. Without pleasure centers and reward pathways in our brains incentivizing our efforts, we might not have sufficient drive to seek out either one. Hunting and gathering take a lot of work. No surprise, then, that our appetites and food cravings are governed in part by the "feel good" messengers in our brains: our bodies' natural cannabinoids, cannabis compounds for a "munchies" effect; endorphins, our own body's natural opioids; the "reward hormone" dopamine; the "happiness hormone" serotonin;[227] and even the love hormone, oxytocin.[228] Dopamine release is such an important motivator of food intake[229] that animals genetically engineered to be unable to make dopamine simply starve themselves to death.[230] Food just doesn't seem to do much for them anymore.

We evolved for millions of years in an environment where sodium was scarce, so a taste for saltiness used to give us a survival advantage, since we need sufficient sodium to live. Calories were sometimes scarce, too, but we didn't need nutrition labels to tell us which foods had more energy. Our taste for sweetness led us to ripe fruit, and our taste for fat drew us to nuts and seeds. The food industry has hijacked these natural drives and turned them against us.

How do we know that the same tactics used to formulate cigarettes to be as addictive as possible have been applied to create ultra-processed foods? From tobacco industry documents themselves.[231] Taste engineers (yes, *taste engineers*) manipulate the salt, sugar, and fat contents of foods to achieve what the industry calls *the bliss point,* the peak of craveability.[232] When owned by tobacco companies, food brands are generally three times more hyperpalatable than comparable brands not under tobacco ownership.[233]

Ultra-processed foods addiction is not recognized as an official diagnosis,[234] but highly processed foods can be considered addictive substances based on established scientific criteria using the same standards established for tobacco products.[235]

Criterion 1 is *compulsive use*, which is clearly the case for highly processed foods.

Criterion 2 is *psychoactivity*, defined as producing "transient alterations in mood that are primarily mediated by effects in the brain." Chocoholics can experience a euphoria rating similar to what is achieved after a smoker is infused with nicotine. Alternatively, when someone is given opioid blockers like Narcan, they eat fewer candies and cookies.[236] This suggests sugar consumption causes the release of endorphins, explaining why more than a hundred randomized controlled studies have found pain-relieving effects of a little sugar water for infants undergoing painful procedures.[237] In contrast, opiate blockers did not affect the intake of an unprocessed, whole-food source of sugar—orange segments in one study—like it did chocolate cookies or, especially, cheese sandwiches.[238]

Criterion 3 is *reinforcing*, meaning we keep wanting to do it, and criterion 4 is *cravings*. Indeed, highly processed foods tend to be the most craved.[239]

There are also two secondary criteria suggested by the Surgeon General's report: *withdrawal symptoms* and *tolerance*, needing a bigger hit to get the same effect.[240] People have reported physical and psychological symptoms reminiscent of tobacco withdrawal when they've attempted to cut down on ultra-processed foods, with symptoms peaking at two to five days and decreasing over the next week or two.[241] This parallels the very time course of withdrawal syndromes for addictive substances.[242]

In terms of tolerance, increased consumption of sugary beverages is associated with a blunted dopamine brain response to a mouthful of sugar.[243] Frequent consumption of ice cream was also found to reduce our brain reward–region responsivity in ways that parallel the tolerance seen in drug addiction.[244]

The field of food addiction is emerging, and not without debate or criticism.[245] Some suggest that food addiction cannot exist because we have to eat,[246] but that's like arguing that alcoholism cannot exist because we have to drink. We have to breathe, too, but we don't have to breathe in tobacco. And, yes, we have to eat, but we don't have to eat junk.

It's certainly true that not all people exhibit an addictive pattern when it comes to ultra-processed products, but the same is true of addictive drugs.[247] For example, only about one in six people who try cocaine goes on to develop a cocaine addiction.[248]

A researcher funded by the largest soda company argued that blaming excessive eating on food addiction risks trivializing "serious addictions."[249] That's exactly what employees of the largest tobacco company said, asserting that labeling smoking as an addiction "minimizes the tragedy of hard-core drug addictions."[250]

The Coca-Cola rep even argued there was a well-documented case of carrot addiction,[251] so we should leave soda alone. And it's actually true. "I just wanted to eat a nice juicy carrot and couldn't stop munching after that," the patient reportedly said.[252] But that has to be the exception that proves the rule. In a study of ultra-processed foods and binge eating, 100% of the foods people binged on were ultra-processed foods.[253] No one was binging on broccoli.

THE NOVA CLASSIFICATION SYSTEM

As I discussed in the Introduction, the NOVA system of food classification categorizes all foods as minimally processed, processed, or ultra-processed.[254] The launch of NOVA's system propelled food processing to the forefront of public health and education.[255] And the backlash began.

Industry Backlash

In response to the increased scrutiny, a small cadre of researchers with declared ties to ultra-processed food manufacturers started pumping out a disproportionate number of articles challenging the legitimacy of the ultra-processed foods concept.[256] For example, researchers funded by two of the largest players in the multitrillion-dollar processed food industry market, Nestlé and Danone,[257] questioned the functionality of the NOVA system. The researchers claimed that overall consistency among evaluators was low,[258] suggesting that identifying ultra-processed foods is akin to when the judge in the famous obscenity case defined hard-core pornography as, "I know it when I see it."[259]

Evaluators largely guessed that commercial orange juice was ultra-processed, for instance, even though 100% fruit juice is considered *minimally* processed in the NOVA system.[260] But just because they didn't know the system doesn't mean the system is invalid. These responses were collected from a survey that enrolled a convenience sample of "evaluators" untrained in NOVA criteria.[261] But people can be trained with just a simple flow chart to see which foods belong in which group.[262] When NOVA was evaluated by trained individuals without industry ties, there was less than 5% disagreement across assessments.[263] The independent researchers concluded: "References used to support claims that Nova lacks clarity almost invariably have authors who are or have been employees of, consultants to, or funded by corporations that produce or market UPF," ultra-processed foods.[264]

The industry grasps at strawmen. "Unknown to most consumers," wrote an employee of an ultra-processed food conglomerate, "even fresh vegetables and fruits are treated with postharvest treatments...."[265] Others point out that processing can sometimes improve the nutritional quality of foods; for example, there is increased bioavailability of the antioxidant lycopene in tomato paste, compared to fresh tomatoes.[266] A professor emeritus of food biotechnology and food process engineering lamented, "Food processing is under severe criticism despite of its 3.3 million years history," citing the invention of stone tools.[267]

The reason these arguments are specious is that food processing itself is not at issue.[268] In the original commentary that started it all, the originator of the NOVA system emphasized that there is nothing wrong with the modification of fresh foods by processing *as such*.[269] He wasn't suggesting we all become raw foodists. The point of the NOVA system is to differentiate between minimally processed foods, processed foods, and ultra-processed industrial formulations that are passed off as food.[270]

Another fallacious argument put forth by Big Food consultants is that adding nutrients to foods makes them ultra-processed. So, for example, if women avoided grain products fortified with folate before conception, their infants might be at increased risk for birth defects. In other words, *think of the children*.[271] But it's simply not true. According to the NOVA system, foods can have added vitamins and minerals and still be considered minimally processed.[272]

A more important question to ask may be *why* do some foods need additional vitamins and minerals? White flour is "enriched" because so much of its nutrition has been stripped away by processing.[273] Ironically, processing can also have the opposite effect. Remember how the polishing of brown rice to white led to the thiamine-deficiency disease beriberi, resulting in the deaths of millions?[274] At the same time, *lack* of processing led to the sickening of millions with the niacin-deficiency disease pellagra[275] (when the step of presoaking corn with alkali was skipped in the production process).[276] Food processing can be good or bad.

The question is: *Can* ultra-*processing be good or bad?*

Another common industry criticism from the likes of candy bar companies is that the science just isn't in yet.[277] Without a randomized controlled trial, how do we *really* know that feeding kids Day-Glo marshmallows for breakfast might not be the best choice? This is reminiscent of the infamous 1994 congressional hearing, where CEOs for the seven largest tobacco companies in America testified under oath that nicotine wasn't addictive and the purported link between cigarettes and lung cancer had yet to be settled.[278]

Robust, randomized, clinical trial data are lacking to support most nutrition recommendations,[279] as diseases can take decades to develop. All we can do is make decisions based on the best available balance of evidence, and that evidence isn't looking very good for ultra-processed foods.

Some NOVA criteria are criticized as being arbitrary. For example, is it fair to judge products based on how many ingredients they have? The NOVA definition of ultra-processed foods has been questioned for its cut-off at five ingredients.[280] Presumably, that number came from Michael Pollan,[281] who NOVA researchers cite as inspiration, but, as with so many industry criticisms, it's simply not true. Ultra-processed foods are described as industrial formulations that *typically* have five or more ingredients, but that's not an absolute rule.[282]

Other charges of arbitrariness seem more grounded. Take coffee, for instance. Though coffee's a far cry from how it's found in nature, it is considered a NOVA 1 food—minimally processed—because the processing method, however industrial, is considered "a traditional processing method."[283] Anything homemade is considered *not* ultra-processed by definition, and certainly some really unhealthy stuff can be made at home.[284] True, the concoctions whipped up in our own kitchens might not have some of the harmful additives and packaging contaminants, but the NOVA scheme is not saying that all *non*-ultra-processed foods are good for us. It's just saying that we should be wary about the ultra-processed ones.

Another critique with some merit is the possibility of unidentified residual confounding, meaning the true cause of disease association may be due to differences that haven't yet been accounted for between those who consume a lot of ultra-processed foods and those who don't. Most studies controlled for obvious factors, like smoking and exercise, but there may be others at play, like age or socio-economic status.[285] At first glance, it might seem that the fact that rates of practically every non-communicable disease are elevated among consumers of ultra-processed foods would strengthen the argument for how bad they are, but if this extends to disease associations that seem implausible, the case would be weakened.

For example, the researchers involved in one large study that found links between the intake of ultra-processed foods and multiple cancers went out of their way to see if intake was also associated with death by accident, since it's hard to imagine how the degree of food processing could contribute to the risk of falling to one's death or drowning.[286] And, indeed: Ultra-processed food consumption was also associated with accidental death.[287] So, perhaps it's less about the food itself and more about the type of people who eat those kinds of foods. Perhaps they live in a way that puts them broadly at risk, like struggling financially or being young and reckless.

However, if you look at the studies on ultra-processed foods and premature death, they all took age into account and nearly all of them considered level of education, income, smoking, and physical activity. Some even controlled for living alone, time spent watching TV, alcohol intake, marital status, or time spent sleeping or snacking. The researchers really did seem to cover their bases. And, even after controlling for all these factors, they still found this association between ultra-processed food consumption and death and disease.[288] So, for accidental death, yes, maybe people who eat a lot of junk also tend not to wear their seatbelts, but the moral to that story is not just to buckle up on your way to the drive-through, but buckle up and consider a trip to the farmer's market instead.

Response to Industry Criticism

I belong to the first generation of U.S. health care professionals in a century to preside over a decline in life expectancy.[289] Could it be because we're gorging ourselves with an ungodly 600 pounds of ultra-processed products per person every year?[290] So-called foods and drinks containing hundreds of novel ingredients to which the human body had never previously been exposed now constitute close to 60% of the diets of American adults and nearly 70% of our children's.[291]

Concern over these kinds of foods is nothing new; I remember my mom keeping sugary cereals and beverages out of the house. A review of resistance efforts noted that she and others "who raised alarm about the encroachment of ultra-processed foods were often labeled, especially by industry and their powerful allies, as 'food faddists' and 'pseudoscientists.'" Dr. Fredrick Stare, the then-chair of nutrition at Harvard University, was among those lobbing such labels on critics of sugar, all while urging a doubling of dietary sugar intake and describing high-sugar cereals as "good food." (You will not be surprised to learn that he received hundreds of thousands of dollars from snack and cereal manufacturers.)[292]

Joan Dye Gussow, one of the great matriarchs of the healthy food movement, wrote: "Those who use old-fashioned methods to achieve...good diets are said to be 'faddists', while the 'rational American' is the one who consumes large quantities of Bac-Os, Tab, Boo-Berry cereal, and hamburger helpers." In response to the first organized protest against the processed food industry, the so-called Nutrition Foundation, a conglomerate led by Coca-Cola, Dow Chemical, General Mills, Kellogg's, and other corporations of their ilk, railed: "This deliberate creation of unwanted anxiety through the dissemination of misinformation concerning our vital basic foods constitutes a glaring breach of public trust and responsibility."[293]

The ultra-processed food industry has maintained its "vice-like grip on the narrative"[294] that there are no good foods or bad foods.[295] When national surveys showed that most American adults agreed with the statement "Nutritionally speaking, I believe there are good foods and bad foods," the American Dietetic Association (ADA, now known as the Academy of Nutrition and Dietetics) responded that "the population was 'mistaken' in their beliefs and needed to be disabused of such notions."[296] That may come as a surprise, but probably less so if you knew the dietitian organization has accepted millions of dollars in corporate contributions from soda and candy bar companies and the like.[297]

Predictably, the ultra-processed foods industry argues that "we must never condemn individual food items but rather should discuss overall diets"[298]— the *all-foods-fit* philosophy.[299] Gussow responded to "the ADA's 'it's all part of a balanced diet' schtick: 'If you tell people there's no difference between a candy bar and an apple, and they already have bad eating habits, what do you think they'll do? There's already a lot of mental justification going on.'"[300]

The bottom line, wrote esteemed nutrition scientist Walter Willett and colleagues, is that "some foods are beneficial for health and others are detrimental. True, an unhealthy food consumed infrequently and in small amounts may do no harm, but this is simply a function of exposure and is also valid for many toxic substances."[301]

We know the food industry cribs straight from the tobacco industry playbook—"supplying misinformation, use of supposedly conflicting evidence, and hiding negative data."[302] In an analysis of food industry submissions to the World Health Organization, most of the claims made did not cite any evidence at all, and two-thirds of those that did came from industry-linked sources, even though most failed to declare conflicts of interest. Overall, of the six claims out of more than a hundred that actually drew on research that was both independent and peer-reviewed, not a single one accurately represented the source.[303]

Should we expect anything different? That's just how the system works,[304] and exploitative industries fight to keep that system in place. Of all the powerful, harmful industries, the ultra-processed food lobby spends the most on lobbying—more than a billion dollars. That's more than Big Tobacco, Big Booze, and the gambling industry (Big Bets?).[305]

It's hardly a secret why companies make and market ultra-processed foods and drinks; they are very profitable. When made with taxpayer-subsidized sugar, the ingredients may cost less than 10% of the retail price.[306] McValue Meal Deal burgers are thanks in part to hundreds of billions of dollars of U.S. federal subsidies for cheap animal feed.[307] Those who resist calls for "heavy-handed" government regulation may not realize those heavy hands are already pressing down the scale on the side of big business.

Industry-funded critics bristle at this kind of talk. Why should it matter *why* a food is being designed and produced?[308] Prioritizing wealth over health has significant real-world consequences. Let's not forget that it was the tobacco industry that originally flooded the market with ultra-processed food.[309] Nowadays, managers of large hedge funds exert substantial influence on the governance of major ultra-processed food corporations in their quest to maximize short-term returns.[310] A former Pepsi CEO rolled out a "good for you" product category in an attempt to "reduce the negative health impact of 'junk food.'" The effort was "met with rancor" by the Board of Directors due to profits plummeting by $349 million.[311]

Note I said *former* CEO.

It's not their fault. Corporations just do what they're set up to do.[312] Their goal is not to make people sick. Their goal is to make people money. "Put simply," concluded a global health institute director, "the enormous commercial success enjoyed by the food industry is now causing what promises to be one of the greatest public health disasters of our time."[313] The bottom line is that these companies may not have our families' best interests at heart.

The industry suggests it is unrealistic to advise people to avoid ultra-processed foods.[314] After all, who has time to cook these days?[315] Those who don't think healthy foods can be convenient have never met an apple.

Some question "abstinence approaches" to ultra-processed foods, but it doesn't have to be all or nothing. There are harm reduction strategies even for people who abuse alcohol, such as avoiding hard liquor and not drinking alone. Similarly, we can split that dessert with a friend or not keep pastries in the house.[316] At the very least, we can not feed junk to kids at school. New York City, for example, successfully eliminated processed meat from its massive public school system.[317] It can be done.

We could also restrict advertising. In 2019, Transport for London implemented restrictions on advertising products high in fat, sugar, and salt on all its subways, buses, trains, and taxis in the city that serve millions every day. That one change in advertising policy alone is estimated to have prevented nearly 100,000 cases of obesity within the subsequent three years, as well as preventing thousands of cases of diabetes and cardiovascular disease.[318]

Is Reformulation the Solution?

In 1945, the American Medical Association's Council on Foods and Nutrition was presented with a new product. Vi-Chocolin was a vitamin-fortified chocolate bar "offered ostensibly as a specialty product of high nutritive value...but in reality intended for promotion to the public as a...vitaminized candy."[319] Surely something like that couldn't happen today? But that seems to be the entire sugary cereal industry's business model. LOADED (frosting-filled) Trix cereal has 12 vitamins and minerals,[320] 50% more than the measly eight found in Marshmallow Froot Loops.[321]

As one medical journal editorial read, "Adding vitamins and minerals to sugary cereals...is worse than useless. The subtle message accompanying such products is that it is safe to eat more."[322] Fruity Pebbles has had "excellent source of vitamin D" emblazoned on its box[323] to create a "nutritional façade" that distracts attention from the fact that we're feeding our kids candy for breakfast.[324]

Concerned about sugar? Not a problem. Cookie Crisp Sprinkles was reformulated to no longer contain 10 grams of sugar but a mere 9 grams per 26-gram serving, so it's now only 35% straight sugar instead of 38%.[325] Reformulation is considered to be an "unobtrusive strategy" by industry, one that "creates the prospect of nutritional improvement without dietary change."[326] The focus is on changing the nutrient profile of a product rather than decreasing its consumption.[327]

Imagine if kids started eating fruit in non-pebbled form!

Reformulation also allows the food and beverage industries to frame themselves as being "part of the solution," similar to how the tobacco industry created and promoted low-tar cigarettes.[328] In an ad for low-tar True brand cigarettes, a young woman sits on the floor in her bellbottoms and clogs, a lit True in her hand. The copy reads: "I thought about all I'd read and said to myself, either quit or smoke True. I smoke True."[329] Many others did, too, inhaling so many so-called light, mild, or low-tar smokes that they earned more than 80% of the market share.[330] Russian Cheetos have 34% less salt, and British Oreos 24% less saturated fat.[331] Anything to keep people from quitting.

Many ultra-processed products try to create a false impression of healthfulness by adding dietary fiber, replacing sugar with artificial sweeteners, or reducing sodium. The tweaks enable manufacturers to make health claims despite their products remaining unhealthy.[332] That's the limit of the market. The invisible hand is more than happy to hand us any kind of junk we want—low-fat junk, low-carb junk, non-GMO organic junk, and—especially ironically—processed paleo junk.[333] They can make money off any fad, except real food.

Shareholders can profit off Funyuns but can't earn much from real onions. Within a narrow scope of commodity components and chemicals, endless reformulations can fit any fashionable flavor of the month, but that's why the ultra-processed food concept is so threatening to the food industry. Non-junk is the one thing they can't make.

Even if the industry could concoct a product that checked all the nutrient profile boxes, it could still be considered an ultra-processed food. Indeed, even without reformulation, about one in eight ultra-processed foods may meet a nutrient profiling system's cut-off for being relatively healthy,[334] but a nutrients-only approach ignores the other potential downsides of ultra-processed foods.[335] Sometimes, being part of the solution makes the problem even worse, like when the switch to partially hydrogenated oils flooded the market with trans fats[336] that may still be killing hundreds of thousands annually.[337]

However, there are reformulations that could make a real, positive difference.[338] For example, removing menthol from cigarettes could potentially reduce their addictiveness enough to allow hundreds of thousands of smokers to quit.[339]

A parallel might be removing caffeine from soda. There's a reason why most of the sugar-sweetened beverages we consume have caffeine added to them. When researchers randomized people to drink the same soda with or without caffeine, the study participants drank 50% more of the caffeinated variety.[340] Given that the consumption of sugar-sweetened beverages may contribute to the deaths of literally hundreds of thousands of people a year,[341] regulators and health professionals should consider increasing the pressure on beverage companies to reformulate their drinks to remove caffeine.[342]

EXCEPTIONS TO THE RULE

The implication that minimally processed foods are healthier than heavily processed foods, which are healthier than ultra-processed foods, is not always the case.

Unprocessed but Unhealthy

Food Compass is a nutrient profiling system[343] that scores foods on a scale from 1 (least healthy) to 100 (most healthy).[344] Figure 4 shows examples of foods scoring a perfect 100 and those scoring the worst, all the way from kale down to cola.[345]

Foods scoring 70 or more are considered foods to be encouraged, scoring 31 to 69 are foods to be moderated, and 30 or less are foods to be minimized.[346] It's easy to understand why more than 90% of ultra-processed foods don't score 70 or higher, but the majority of the least processed foods don't make the cut either.[347] The reason is that animal foods like eggs, milk, and fresh meat are considered minimally processed. Although the NOVA 1 category of unprocessed or minimally processed foods includes a lot of whole plant foods—the foundation for healthy diets[348]—the animal foods drag down the average Food Compass score.[349]

Figure 5 is from an analysis of 8,000 foods. As you can see, nearly all of the minimally processed plant foods average 70 or higher, compared to none of the minimally processed animal foods.[350]

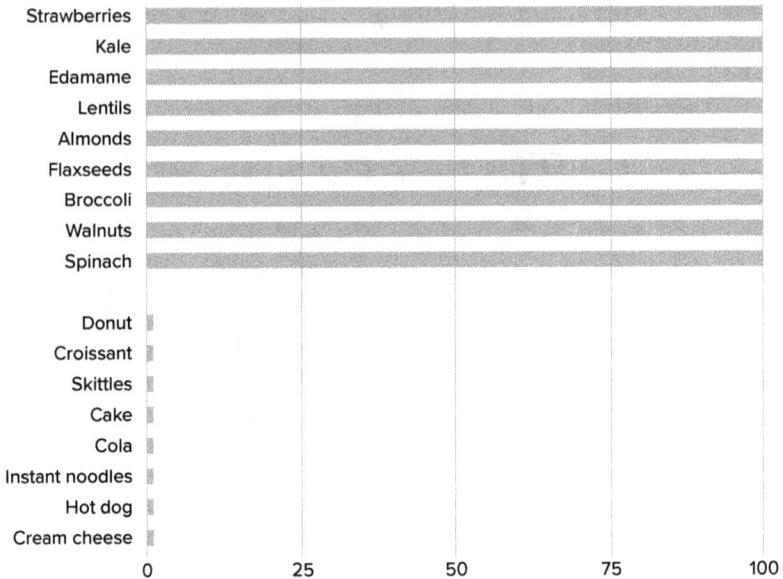

**Examples of Best and Worst Foods
Scored by Food Compass**

Figure 4

There are reviews of the adverse effects of ultra-processed foods that make the leap to the non-sequitur "eggs, meat, milk, etc. may render broad public health benefits,"[351] but that doesn't make sense. Following that logic, butter is good for us because margarine is bad. Just because a biscuit is bad, doesn't mean brisket is good.

The American Heart Association makes this point in its latest dietary guidance document, advising us to "choose minimally processed foods instead of ultra-processed foods" and, at the same time, emphasizing that we should eat foods low in cholesterol and saturated fat.[352] As an editorial in the *British Medical Journal* cautioned, "Recommendations to avoid ultra-processed food may...give the impression that foods that are not ultra-processed are healthy and can be freely consumed. This is problematic—for example, the [leading public health authorities] IARC and WCRF have concluded that red meat (categorized by the Nova system as

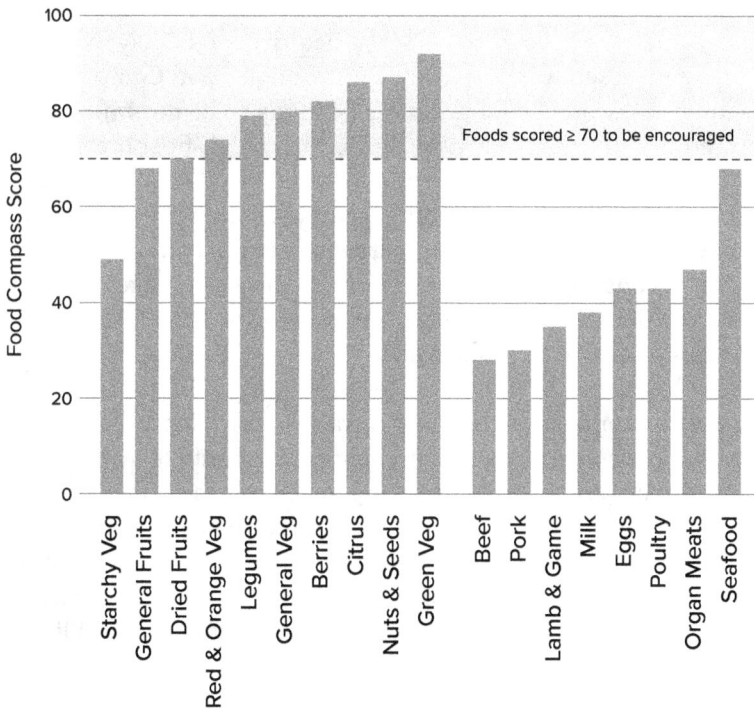

Average Food Compass Scores for Minimally Processed Plant and Animal Foods

Food Compass Score

Foods scored ≥ 70 to be encouraged

Starchy Veg, General Fruits, Dried Fruits, Red & Orange Veg, Legumes, General Veg, Berries, Citrus, Nuts & Seeds, Green Veg, Beef, Pork, Lamb & Game, Milk, Eggs, Poultry, Organ Meats, Seafood

Figure 5

'unprocessed or minimally processed')...probably increases the risk of bowel cancer,"[353] the leading cancer killer of nonsmokers in the United States.[354,355]

Unprocessed meat also appears to increase the risk of bladder cancer, breast cancer, endometrial cancer, esophageal cancer, head and neck cancer, lung cancer, lymphoma, stomach cancer, and death from all cancers combined.[356] Beyond cancer, unprocessed meat consumption has also been associated with a significantly increased risk of type 2 diabetes, heart disease, high blood pressure, and stroke.[357] Unprocessed does not necessarily mean unproblematic.

Ultra-Processed but Healthy?

Just as there are minimally processed foods that aren't the best choices, some ultra-processed foods aren't the worst. The American Heart Association guidelines specify that "some healthy foods may exist within the ultra-processed food category."[358] Although Food Compass categorized most ultra-processed products as foods to be minimized, nearly 7% scored as being relatively healthful.[359] Many high-fiber breakfast cereals, for example, may be "adversely classified by NOVA" as, technically, they are ultra-processed, but reducing our consumption of them "would be expected to exacerbate [our] already low fibre intakes"—at least so argues a consultant for Nestlé,[360] which proudly makes candy bar–flavored cereals[361] so you can "start your day with 14g of whole grains," encourages an ad for KitKat cereal.[362]

Bread is often touted[363] as a healthy ultra-processed food[364] and an example of why we should not make sweeping statements to avoid all things ultra-processed. Whole-grain bread is a major source of fiber,[365] but bread is also a major source of sodium,[366] considered to be humanity's leading dietary risk factor for death.[367] Industry consultants created an entire ultra-processed foods menu that purportedly conformed with most dietary guidelines; even they couldn't get the sodium to fall in line.[368]

There are a variety of no-salt-added breads on the market,[369] and some of them are hardly processed at all. One even has only two ingredients: organic rye kernels and water.[370] But most packaged breads are ultra-processed, containing such additives as preservatives, colorings, emulsifiers, and dough conditioners, some of which may be toxic, like azodicarbonamide, which is banned in Europe.[371] Another is potassium bromate, which, having been deemed a potential human carcinogen, is banned in Europe, the United Kingdom, Canada, China, Australia, India, Nigeria,[372] and many other countries, though not the United States.[373] Thanks to the California Food Safety Act, though, it will be banned at least in that state as of 2027.[374]

If packaged bread is the best example industry can come up with of a healthy food getting unfairly caught in the ultra-processed category crossfire, it isn't looking too good for ultra-processed foods, especially when we can get our whole grains from a non-KitKat-flavored food like oatmeal.[375]

Ultra-Processed Foods That Are Healthier Than Processed Foods

pH Levels of Various Flavors of Sparkling Waters

BRAND AND FLAVOR	pH
Bubly Grapefruit	3.86
Bubly Lime	3.87
Bubly Cherry	3.89
Bubly Pineapple	4.06
LaCroix Pamplemousse	4.71
LaCroix Lemon	4.79
LaCroix Lime	4.80
LaCroix Pure	4.80
LaCroix Berry	4.83
Perrier Strawberry	5.43
Perrier Pink Grapefruit	5.46
Perrier	5.47
Perrier Lemon	5.47

Prolonged exposure to beverages below 5.2 may be erosive to dental enamel.

Figure 6

There are some genuinely healthful ultra-processed foods, like Uncle Sam Cereal (sadly discontinued after a century in 2024 after Post bought it) or certain no-salt-added tomato sauces, which score high on multiple nutrient profile scorings but are considered ultra-processed[376] because of additives like barley malt[377] and citric acid, respectively.[378] A no-salt sauce with citric acid would certainly be better than a salty citric acid–free sauce.[379] It would be an example of an ultra-processed product that could be better than one merely processed with the addition of salt, but that still wouldn't necessarily be a case of an ultra-processed product that would be better than a *minimally* processed version without the added salt, sugar, or additives.

An unsweetened drink like LaCroix,[380] ultra-processed because it's "naturally essenced" (whatever that means), is certainly healthier than most NOVA 4 ultra-processed beverages like Coca-Cola[381] and NOVA 3 processed drinks like beer. It's also healthier than a NOVA 1 beverage like whole milk. (Whole milk, along with beer, is classified by the prestigious Beverage Guidance Panel as one of the least healthy beverages, complete with a recommendation to consume zero ounces a day.[382]) That said, LaCroix still doesn't beat out plain water, since sparkling water tends to be more likely to dip below the cut-off for acidity (5.2 pH) that may be harmful to our tooth enamel over time.[383] (If you drink sparkling water, I encourage you to rinse your mouth with plain water afterwards to protect your dental enamel.) Figure 6 shows the measured pH levels of various flavors of sparkling waters.[384]

So, it comes down to "the eternal question" in the field of nutrition: *Instead of what?*[385] Is LaCroix good for us? Compared to Coke, yes; compared to plain water, no. That's the question we need to ask when critics fear that, in the demonization of ultra-processed foods, we might be throwing out the baby with the bathwater.[386]

Ultra-Processed Foods That Are Healthier Than Unprocessed Foods?

Infant formula is often held up as an example[387] of an ultra-processed product that is health-promoting, but *instead of what?* The less-processed food it's meant to replace—human breast milk—is far superior. (Whenever possible, breast is best, as there is "extensive evidence of important health risks" related to using infant formula.[388]) Are there any instances in which the baby-with-the-bathwater concern holds legitimacy? Any examples of ultra-processed foods that are actually healthier than the foods they were designed to replace?

What about plant-based milks and plant-based meats? They're ultra-processed.[389] If justifiable ultra-processed food phobia slowed the acceptance of plant-based eating, that could have global health implications[390]—and, indeed, the level of processing does appear to be a significant reason many people are avoiding plant-based substitutes.[391] However, this preclusion is only a public health problem if these products are healthier than conventional animal products.

Unsurprisingly, those who work for the ultra-processed plant-based industry think their products are healthier.[392] Skeptics contend that this argument "appears to be part of the 'planting doubt' playbook"—pun intended—"which aims to exonerate manufacturers from other public health concerns" about ultra-processed products like Twinkies.[393] That is a common strategy of corporate actors who argue that *their* products are the exception and being unfairly misclassified or confused with *genuinely* harmful foods.[394] In response to a call by Big Soy consultants to revise the concept of ultra-processed foods to avoid targeting plant-based alternatives,[395] a public health nutrition professor emphasized the "need for particular scrutiny of claims made by researchers associated with ultra-processed food manufacturers."[396]

"It is strange that in claiming they are arguing for healthy and sustainable diets," the professor continued, they "appear to be more concerned with challenging the UPF concept than promoting already available non-UPF foods," like beans. He concluded by demanding "close scrutiny" of the integrity of the industry-affiliated researchers' claims.[397] The industry consultants replied in a letter to the editor of the journal, accusing the professor of "classic ad hominem reasoning" for pointing out their industry affiliations instead of focusing on their argument.[398] Their accusation may have carried more weight had that list of affiliations not been twice as long as their entire letter.[399]

Their more substantive response was that they, of course, wholeheartedly support increased intake of whole plant foods. "However, the products in question are designed to replace meat and dairy products not legumes and nuts. Therefore, the critical comparisons are between hamburgers and soya burgers and cows' milk and soyamilk"—that is, with the foods the plant-based alternatives were designed to replace.[400]

The primary objective of ultra-processed "fake" foods is to imitate "real" foods. Think strawberry Pop-Tarts trying to mimic actual strawberries.[401] When you start with a food with a perfect Food Compass score of 100, like strawberries, the only way to go is down.[402] So, real fruit is better than Froot Loops' *Fruity Shaped* marshmallows.[403] But when the "real" food is dairy or unprocessed, processed, or ultra-processed meat, as you can see in Figure 7, there is a lot of room for improvement.[404]

Room for Improvement

	Food Compass Score
Strawberries, raw	100
Cheddar cheese	26
Pork chop, stewed	25
Bacon, cooked	24
Hot dog	1

Figure 7

EVALUATING PLANT-BASED MEATS

Professor Monteiro, the originator of the ultra-processed concept, proposed 16 different mechanisms for how ultra-processed foods may contribute to the risk of death and disease.[405] Typically, ultra-processed foods not only have a junkier nutrient profile than the foods they are designed to replace, but they also tend to be higher in calorie density, have a softer texture (think Wonder Bread), a degraded food matrix, and missing phytonutrients. They may also contain industrial contaminants like AGEs, harmful additives, and chemicals that leach in from their packaging. The displacement of whole foods and addictive qualities can lead to calorie excess and weight gain, which in turn can contribute to metabolic disorders like diabetes. What's more, ultra-processed foods may damage our gut microbiome, cause low-grade systemic inflammation, impair our artery function, and lead to oxidative stress (an excess of free radicals).

How does plant-based meat compare to conventional meat on all these metrics?

Nutritional Quality

"Are Plant-Based Meat Alternative Products Healthier Than the Animal Meats They Mimic?" asked the title of a nutrition journal review.[406] Let's see what the Food Compass nutrient profiling system scoring from 1 to 100 has to say. If you remember, it suggests actively encouraging consumption of foods scoring 70 and above, actively minimizing intake of foods scoring 30 or below, and consuming in moderation anything scoring in between.

Rather than encourage/moderate/minimize messaging, in nutrition, it's helpful to use the "compared to what" approach.[407] How healthy is something compared to what might otherwise be eaten?

Counterfactual Food

Figure 8 shows the dozen ultra-processed meatless alternatives that were scored.[408]

As you can see in Figure 8, in every case, the plant-based meat scored healthier than its closest conventional meat match—and sometimes by a large margin. Nearly all plant-based meats scored at least twice as high.[409] By choosing the meatless equivalent, in most cases, we would move out of the foods-to-be-minimized range into, at least, the foods to be eaten in moderation.

Now, better than chicken-free chicken (score: 54) would be chickpeas (score: 90), and better than soyburgers (score: 60) would be soybeans (score: 100),[410] but the choice on the Burger King menu is between a Whopper and an Impossible Whopper, not between a Whopper and steamed edamame. (Of course, there is a third choice—not ending up at Burger King in the first place.)

Health Star Rating and Nutri-Score

Figure 8 includes two other nutrient scoring systems for comparison. The Health Star Rating[411] was developed by the Australian government to rate foods from ½ star to 5 stars, with the more stars, the better.[412] It was designed, as it should be, to compare similar foods to help individuals make healthier choices,[413] but foods that rate 2 stars or less can be thought of as having an unhealthy profile, while those scoring 3.5 or more suggesting a healthy profile.[414]

As you can see in Figure 8, most of the meatless options made the cut for being considered healthy.[415] More importantly, they scored better than the conventional meat equivalents in nearly every case. And, in most cases, the plant-based option flipped the script from unhealthy to healthy.[416]

Nutritional Scoring of Ultra-Processed Plant-Based Meat

	Food Compass Score	Health Star Rating	Nutri-Score
Breaded Meatless Chicken	68	4.5	A
Chicken Tenders or Strips	34	2	D
Luncheon Slices (Meatless Beef, Chicken, Salami, or Turkey)	63	3.5	C
Luncheon Meat	16	3	D
Meatless Meatballs	62	4	A
Meatballs with Sauce	19	2	D
Meatless Hot Dog	61	4	A
Hot Dog	1	1	E
Meatless Breakfast Link	60	2	D
Sausage	8	1	E
Vegetarian Burger	60	4	A
Ground Beef Patty	26	2	D
Meatless Bacon	57	1	D
Bacon	24	0.5	E
Meatless Chicken	54	4	B
Baked or Broiled Skinless Chicken Breast	46	4	B
Soyburger with Cheese	30	3.5	C
Whopper with Cheese	15	2	D
Chili with Meat Substitute	85	5	A
Chili with Meat	29	3	C
Meatless Swiss Steak with Gravy	65	3.5	B
Swiss Steak	44	4	A
Meat Substitute Sandwich Spread	89	4	A
Potted Meat	2	1.5	D

Figure 8

Nutri-Score is a five-tiered, color-coded system used in Europe to denote overall nutritional quality from *A* (best) to *E* (worst).[417] The food industry hates it, which is usually a good sign.[418] As shown in Figure 8, most of the meatless options scored an *A* or a *B*, and most of the conventional meats scored a *D* or an *E*. Most importantly, the plant-based alternatives rated healthier in almost every case.[419] This suggests that plant-based meats may indeed be the rare case in which ultra-processed products are healthier than the minimally processed products they were designed to replace.

2,000 Products Compared

Only a handful of ultra-processed plant-based products made it into the Food Compass database. About 100 were tested in Canada, though, and researchers reached the same conclusion: The overall nutritional qualities of plant-based meats were healthier than their animal-based counterparts. The same was also found in Australia, Italy, the United Kingdom, and Sweden.[420]

In the United Kingdom, researchers looked at more than 200 plant-based meats and found that, overall, they had a better nutrient profile than their animal-based meat equivalents, which were about three times more likely to fall into the worst category based on the UK's Nutrient Profiling Model.[421] UK plant-based products also scored better than their animal-based counterparts using the Nutri-Score system.[422]

When more than 200 products in Italy were Nutri-Scored, results clearly showed a higher number of plant-based meats grading better than meat options.[423] About a hundred products in the Australian and New Zealand markets were analyzed, and the Health Star Ratings of plant-based sausages scored better than meat-based ones, plant-based burgers better than meat burgers, ground meat was comparable, plant-based bacon scored much higher than pig-based, and all categories of plant-based poultry alternatives edged out chicken products.[424]

When more than 300 plant-based meats in Brazil were Nutri-Scored, researchers found that about 80% scored at least an *A*, *B*, or *C*, while the opposite was seen with conventional meat products—80% got the worst scores, *D* or *E*.[425] Nutri-Scoring more than 400 plant-based meats in Spain had similar findings, with most meat alternatives scoring *A* or *B* and most conventional meats scoring *D* or *E*.[426]

In Germany, more than 700 plant-based meats were scored. That is a lot of veggie schnitzel! Using a nutritional quality measure that compares the levels of harmful components, plant-based meats similarly scored better.[427]

Overall, a 2024 systematic review identified nine studies that assessed meats and their comparable meat-free alternatives for healthfulness using nutritional scoring. All of them—nine out of nine—occasionally found comparable scores for individual categories, but they mostly showed meat alternatives scoring better.[428]

100,000 Cancers and Other Diseases Prevented Per Serving

Based on their nutrient profiles, plant-based meats would be expected to substantially reduce the risks of a variety of chronic diseases, including heart disease, stroke, and cancer. Specifically, risk of these killer diseases would be expected to fall by about 3% per daily serving swap.[429] That means that nationwide in the United States, for example, replacing animal-based meat with plant-based meat just once daily could potentially prevent more than 100,000 cases of heart disease, stroke, or cancer in the country every year. It's hard to get people to go all kale and quinoa overnight, but a veggie burger shouldn't be as difficult.

The estimated dramatic drop in disease was based on the generally healthier nutritional qualities of plant-based meat compared to regular meat, such as less saturated fat and more fiber.[430] Just because plant-based meats are nutritionally superior, though, doesn't mean that they're out of the woods. Nutrient content was just one of 16 factors potentially linking ultra-processed foods to harm.[431]

Beyond Nutrient Profile

Plant-based meats are the ultra-processed exception in terms of nutritional quality, scoring as healthier than the foods they were designed to replace, but are plant-based meats also exceptional when it comes to the 15 other factors?

Calorie Density

Ultra-processed foods typically tend to be worse when it comes to calorie density, but the opposite is true for plant-based meat. A 2024 systematic review found that, in nearly 90% of comparison studies, calorie density was either significantly lower among the meat-free meats or about the same.[432] So, plant-based meats are the ultra-processed exception when it comes to calorie density, too.[433]

Texture

The softer texture of typical ultra-processed foods allows for less chewing and a faster eating speed. However, plant-based meats are designed to have the same texture as conventional meats. In the largest public sensory analysis of plant-based meats, with more than a thousand people comparing dozens of products, the texture of the plant-based meats most commonly matched the texture of animal-based meat, with the texture of plant-based chicken nuggets actually exceeding that of the chicken-based chicken nuggets.[434] So, switching from conventional chicken nuggets to plant-based ones could have both health[435] and gustatory benefits.[436] Either way, adverse texture change is another property that may plague typical ultra-processed foods but doesn't apply to most ultra-processed meat alternatives.[437]

Food Matrix

The degradation of the physical structure of foods leads to the formation of "acellular" nutrients.[438] As previously noted, the cell walls of plants are made of fiber[439] and physically encapsulate intracellular nutrients, such as fat, starch, sugar, and protein.[440] Since we can't break down fiber, intact plant cell walls that miss our molars prevent the release of those nutrients early in the digestive process. When they reach the colon, our fiber-feeding good bacteria break open those cell walls and release the nutrients to feed our microbiome. But when plants are processed into vegetable oil, fruit juice, sugar, or flour, the nutrients can be rendered *acellular*, ripping them out of their cell walls.[441] So, matrix degradation is certainly an issue between ultra-processed meat analogs and *whole* plant foods, but not between plant-based meats and the animal products they were designed to replace,[442] as animal cells don't have any cell walls to begin with. Without fiber, the cell membranes that wrap animal cells are breached early on in our digestive system, depriving our microbiome of benefit.

Phytonutrients and Antioxidants

Another downside of typical ultra-processed foods is missing phytonutrients. Also known as *phytochemicals*, phytonutrients may contribute to the maintenance of good health through their antioxidant, anti-inflammatory, and anti-cancer effects.[443] By definition, phytonutrients are produced only by plants; *phyto* is from the Greek word for "plant." Thousands have been identified, and the processing of plant foods may cause a hundredfold drop in their phytonutrient content.[444] In contrast, when plants are processed through animals (i.e., when animals eat plants), up to 100% of the phytonutrients may be lost. So, it's not surprising that, when plant-based meat was compared to meat even from grass-fed animals, researchers found that many phytonutrients were missing entirely from the grass-fed meat.[445] So, when it comes to phytonutrient content, ultra-processed plant-based meat once again wins out.[446]

The grass-fed meat industry boasts that its products have more phytonutrients than meat from animals raised on conventional feedlot operations,[447] but the levels pale in comparison to plants. For example, it's true that, compared to grain-fed cattle, cows eating green leafy grasses have higher levels of the plant-based antioxidants vitamin E and beta carotene in their blood,[448] which translates to more phytonutrients in the meat—up to twice as much vitamin E and about seven times as much beta carotene than conventionally raised cattle. But almonds have more than a hundred times more vitamin E and a single carrot can have a thousand times more beta carotene. Similarly, grass-fed meat may have 2.5 milligrams of vitamin C instead of the 1.5 milligrams in feedlot meat,[449] but an orange has 50 times more.[450]

Researchers have found that grass-fed beef may have as much as 50% more antioxidant power than grain-fed,[451] though other studies did not find any difference or saw even less antioxidant power in meat from pasture-raised animals.[452] But, for the sake of argument, let's say that grass-fed meat did in fact have 50% more antioxidants. In an analysis of the total antioxidant content of thousands of different foods, animal-based foods average

18 antioxidant units (in modified FRAP assay daμmols). So, at 50% more, grass-fed meat may have as much as 27 units, but plant-based foods average more than 1,000 antioxidant units.[453]

Plant-based meats may pale in comparison to the whole plants they may have been made with, but they still average twice as much antioxidant power as the meats they were designed to replace.[454]

Advanced Glycation End-Products

The advanced glycation end-products acronym *AGE* was chosen intentionally.[455] As you may remember from the Processing Contaminants section, AGEs are heat-induced pro-aging toxins involved in nearly every age-related disease.[456] How do the levels in plant-based meats compare?

The largest, most cited database of AGEs in foods includes nine meat burgers and nine plant-based ones. All the meat burgers have AGE levels in the thousands, while all the plant-based burgers are in the hundreds or lower. The average AGE content of meat burgers exceeds 6,000, compared to an average of less than 200 in the plant-based burgers—30 times lower.[457] The thought is that naturally occurring phytonutrients in plants may act as inhibitors against the formation of toxicants, thus improving the safety of meat-free meat.[458]

However, four newer but smaller studies using a more precise method of analysis called *mass spectrometry* found more ambivalent results: One study showed AGE levels higher in the one plant-based burger tested,[459] a second study showed the opposite,[460] a third study found higher levels of one AGE and lower levels of another,[461] and a fourth study found two to three times higher levels of both types of AGEs in beef patties compared to plant-based meats.[462]

Overall, when it comes to AGEs, plant-based meats are once again the exception to the rule that ultra-processed products are necessarily worse than the less-processed foods they were meant to replace. The meatless meats were either superior—30 times better—or about the same when it came to AGE levels, depending on the analysis used.

There are other heat-induced toxins, such as furosine, which may damage kidney and liver cells.[463] It was found at comparable levels in meat and plant-based burgers.[464] Another is acrylamide.

Acrylamide

The food processing contaminant acrylamide is formed by the high, dry heating of mainly starchy foods.[465] Even after decades of research, whether it causes cancer is still an open question. As always, it's better to be safe than sorry.[466]

Plant-based meat can average up to about 70 micrograms of acrylamide per kilogram.[467,468] Those levels are considered "low"[469] when compared to potato chips and french fries, the major dietary sources of acrylamide, which can exceed 1,000 micrograms.[470] But saying something isn't as bad as a french fry isn't saying very much. In Europe, benchmark targets aim to get acrylamide levels in french fries below 500 and baby food below 40, but those are based on what's thought to be achievable, not necessarily what's optimal.[471] If one were to develop a tolerable daily intake, a conservative first approach might be 2.6 micrograms per kilogram of body weight or about 200 micrograms a day as the safety limit for the average-weight American.[472]

At 70 micrograms per kilogram, a typical quarter-pound serving of plant-based meat would contain about 7 micrograms.[473] The average daily intake from foods in general is around 20, so we could eat an additional 25 veggie burgers a day before exceeding the proposed tolerable dose.

Ideally, though, we wouldn't eat hardly any,[474] which is how much raw ground beef can have.[475] However, the fairer comparison is burger to burger, and, in that case, both animal- and plant-based burgers have been reported to have similar levels. So, it's doubly ironic that meat industry–funded lobbyists condemn plant-based products as carcinogenic because of acrylamide in full-page ads showing a skull and crossbones on a package of plant-based bacon. Not only may meat contain the same amount, but the expert consensus is that real bacon actually causes cancer.[476]

Heterocyclic Amines and Polycyclic Aromatic Hydrocarbons

Heterocyclic amines are "poisonous compounds" that are formed when meat is heated. Even trace amounts may cause serious diseases like cancer. Components of muscle, like creatine, are necessary for the formation of the most common and most concerning heterocyclic amines,[477] so we shouldn't expect any in plant-based meats. However, at high enough temperatures, other heterocyclic amines can be created regardless of the presence of muscle.[478] How do the levels compare? There have been four studies to date.

The first published study found none of the four heterocyclic amines tested in plant-based burgers, which helps explain why fried soy burgers were up to 250 times less mutagenic, less DNA-damaging, than fried beef patties. However, the plant-based burgers were patties of tempeh, a fermented whole soy food, and may not have been ultra-processed.[479]

An analysis of an ultra-processed soy burger versus a beef burger found none of one heterocyclic amine in the plant-based burger and similar levels of two others.[480] The third study found less than half as many heterocyclic amines in plant-based burgers,[481] and the final study found their levels to be far lower in plant-based products than in conventional meats.[482] Even the highest level of the most carcinogenic heterocyclic amine found in plant-based products was 25 times lower than what's found in cooked chicken.[483]

The other major cooked meat carcinogen is polycyclic aromatic hydrocarbons, or PAHs.[484] There appears to be only a single study comparing levels in conventional meat and plant-based meat, and it found that PAH levels in plant-based meat were about four to five times lower than in animal-based meat.[485]

Harmful Additives

Meat can cause cancer.[486] According to the prestigious International Agency for Research on Cancer (IARC), processed meat—bacon, ham, hot dogs, lunch meat, sausage, and the like—is a group 1 carcinogen, meaning that the science is in that it causes cancer in humans, whereas something like a steak is only "probably carcinogenic to humans."[487]

In addition to the heterocyclic amines and polycyclic aromatic hydrocarbons, there is strong evidence that the formation of *n-nitroso compounds* like nitrosamines also contribute to cancer risk.[488] N-nitroso compounds are carcinogens that can form inside our gut when we eat meat or already come preformed in nitrite-preserved (cured) meats.[489] Even so-called uncured processed meat labeled as having "no nitrites added" is contaminated. On the label, you'll see an asterisk next to the "no nitrites added" that points to a disclaimer reading along the lines of "except those naturally occurring in cultured celery powder."[490]

The nitrates in celery are fermented into nitrites, so adding it to uncured processed meat is just an underhanded way of adding nitrites. Even meat scientists admit the "no nitrites added" ruse may be viewed as "incorrect at best or deceptive at worst."[491] Since plant-based meat doesn't require nitrite additives (used to prevent botulism from meat),[492] this is another example of how ultra-processed plant-based meats can be less harmful than the less-processed meats they're meant to replace.[493]

There is also evidence that heme iron may play a role in the connection between meat consumption and colorectal cancer.[494] That form of iron is concentrated in muscle meat but also found in the roots of soybean plants[495] and can be churned out to make the Impossible Burger possible.[496] This raises a concern unique among plant-based meats about Impossible Foods beef products.[497] Other cancer authorities consider the evidence linking heme iron and cancer to be more limited.[498] For an in-depth look into this controversy, see my four-part video series starting with see.nf/heme. Regardless, however bad the heme iron in Impossible may be, it wouldn't be worse than the heme in meat.[499]

Is the Emulsifying Food Additive Methylcellulose Harmful?

In one of the largest studies conducted to date that checked the ingredients lists of thousands of products, researchers found that the average number of additives in red meat products, poultry products, and plant-based meat products, whether vegan or not, is not that different.[500] The question then becomes: *What is being added?*

Up to three-quarters of plant-based meats contain thickeners or emulsifiers, perhaps most commonly *methylcellulose*,[501] which is sometimes added to conventional meat, too, including whole cuts.[502] Used as a common thickening agent in foods since the 1940s, methylcellulose[503] is considered safe for all animal species,[504] including humans, but that's also been said about *carboxy*methylcellulose, whose safety is seriously being questioned.[505]

There is growing evidence that suggests emulsifiers might be playing a role in the rapid increase in the incidence of chronic inflammatory diseases over the last three-quarters of a century.[506] The original study that raised the alarm was on carboxymethylcellulose, which causes bacterial overgrowth and intestinal inflammation in mice.[507] Since then, rodent models have shown that emulsifiers like carboxymethylcellulose and polysorbate 80 may induce colitis,[508] accelerate the development of type 1 diabetes,[509] exacerbate the development of intestinal tumors,[510] promote the development of colon cancer,[511] exacerbate food allergies,[512] and promote metabolic disorders[513] and even mental disorders that can[514] affect the subsequent generation. When exposed to these emulsifiers during pregnancy and lactation, mice appear to pass on to their offspring the metabolic impairments, cognition deficits, and anxiety-like traits, even though their progeny were never themselves directly exposed.[515]

Detrimental effects of emulsifiers may be due to alterations of the gut's mucus lining[516] or by direct, pro-inflammatory targeting of the intestinal microbiome.[517] In many cases, antibiotics can reverse emulsifier-induced effects,[518] and the effects of emulsifier consumption can be eliminated under microbiome-free conditions. Emulsifier-induced problems may also be spread through fecal transplants between animals, again demonstrating the role of the microbiome. Gut bugs can even just be mixed with emulsifiers in a petri dish and, when transplanted, recapitulate many of the negative effects.[519]

All of this led the International Organization for the Study of Inflammatory Bowel Disease to recommend that patients with IBD limit their intake of carboxymethylcellulose, polysorbate 80, and other such additives, while acknowledging this is based on a very low level of evidence, predominantly from animal models.[520] But that was before a human study showed that, indeed, there were detrimental impacts to those randomized to being covertly given carboxymethylcellulose,[521] apparently through a similar microbiome mechanism.[522]

Another randomized controlled trial also found human harm from *carrageenan*, another common binder used in both conventional and plant-based meats,[523] and a cross-over trial in which people were randomized to lower or higher emulsifier diets found significant yet paradoxical gut function effects.[524] The bottom line is that we can no longer assume emulsifiers are necessarily safe.

This is especially the case with carboxymethylcellulose, for which we now have human evidence of harm that it "may be contributing to increased prevalence of an array of chronic inflammatory diseases by altering the gut microbiome...."[525]

However, carboxymethylcellulose is not the same as methylcellulose, the ingredient commonly found in the plant-based meats. Methylcellulose is considered so safe that it's taken by the spoonful as a bulk-forming laxative.[526] That's what's in Citrucel,[527] which trademarked methylcellulose[528] as "smartfiber."[529] But, just because it's called safe and smart doesn't necessarily make it so.

A 2024 review of all the experimental evidence on the harm of emulsifiers in animals, humans, and test tubes noted many studies on carboxymethylcellulose and a variety of other emulsifiers, but none on methylcellulose.[530] There have been two population studies linking specific emulsifiers with human diseases,[531] but, in both cases, methylcellulose was consumed so infrequently that it wasn't specifically investigated.[532]

Since dietary emulsifiers may cause problems irrespective of their origin, one might consider methylcellulose guilty until proven innocent.[533] When 20 different emulsifiers were tested in vitro, 18 of the 20 seemed to cause problems.[534] So, although not all were pro-inflammatory, 90% were. Methylcellulose wasn't included in that research, but I was finally able to find one study looking into it.

Mice were given a toxic substance to induce inflammation in their colons. While some fibers like Metamucil helped, methylcellulose made matters worse, at around 10 times the concentration we see in plant-based meat. Does this mean it's necessarily harmful in humans? No. In fact, and as we'll see in the Gut Microbiome section, all the studies that looked at the effects of replacing conventional meat with plant-based meat showed microbiome *benefits*. Might that have just been because of the reduced meat intake? Surprisingly, vegetarians who eat plant-based meat appear to have *lower* rates of irritable bowel syndrome than those who don't eat plant-based meat, which reassuringly suggests that, at least using that metric, the emulsifiers don't seem to be a problem.[535]

No discussion of additives in plant-based meats would be complete without discussing the tara flour debacle.[536] The meal delivery service Daily Harvest introduced French Lentil and Leek Crumble, a high-protein frozen food.[537] It listed six simple ingredients: lentils, butternut squash, hemp seeds, quinoa, cremini mushrooms, and tara.[538] Tara is a new plant-based protein ingredient from the seeds of a South American tree.[539] *Tara* means "flat" in the local language, referring to its flat seeds, the starchy part of which is processed to generate tara gum,[540] which is considered safe for human consumption. All the germ of the seed is left over,[541] though, and its disposal costs money, so it was fed to livestock. Why not grind it into tara protein powder and feed it to people[542] instead? What could go wrong?

Consumers reported horrible abdominal pain, drenching sweats, and intractable nausea, vomiting, and diarrhea. The tragic irony, of course, was that the people were choosing the plant-based crumble because they wanted to eat more healthfully.[543] There were also serious cases of liver injury.[544,545,546]

In all, hundreds of individuals fell ill. While there were no deaths, more than 100 people were hospitalized.[547] Investigators determined that tara flour was the most likely culprit, after another product—a "superfood" smoothie—also tried marketing tara powder to the protein-obsessed. It turns out tara contains a toxic compound called *baikiain* that inhibits an antioxidant enzyme, causing liver injury in a manner analogous to a Tylenol overdose.[548] Some people are more genetically predisposed to be affected than others, similar to how some are born with a genetic defect making them unable to eat fava beans.[549]

Daily Harvest recalled its French Lentil and Leek Crumble,[550] but it took a full year before businesses were told to stop using tara flour by the government of Canada (where the smoothie incident had happened)[551] and two years before the U.S. FDA stripped tara flour of its Generally Recognized As Safe status.[552] How did it get recognized as safe in the first place? Unbelievably, it's up to companies to determine the safety of their own products. That's how new food additives can enter the market with zero independent safety review. That's also how trans fats were able to stay on the market for decades,[553] which, as we've discussed, continue to kill hundreds of thousands of people a year.[554]

In the absence of FDA action, states including California have banned certain food additives, and lawmakers in Illinois and New York have recently proposed similar bans.[555] But, this all underscores how poorly regulated food additives are, leading to the potential for unintended consequences of novel ingredients.[556]

Trans fats are only the tenth leading dietary risk factor for mortality on our planet, though. The leading dietary risk factor for death is the excess intake of sodium.[557] So, the most harmful additive in plant-based meats may be, ironically, the most traditional: salt.

Is Plant-Based Meat Worth Its Salt?

Salt is one of the most common ingredients in plant-based meats.[558] Of course, it's also one of the most frequently used ingredients in conventional meat processing—and not just for processed meat products.[559] While pizza is the number one source of sodium for kids and bread for older Americans, one reason chicken is the number one source of sodium for U.S. adults aged 19 through 50[560] is because injecting saltwater into raw chicken has been a widespread practice in the poultry industry since the 1970s. It results in raw chicken breasts reaching 400 milligrams or more of sodium—six times more than they'd naturally have.[561]

Do ultra-processed plant-based meats have more, less, or the same amount of sodium? It varies geographically. In Canada, a study of about a hundred meat substitutes found them to have significantly less sodium, which is one of the reasons they were found to have a better overall nutritional quality.[562] A similar study in the UK also found meat alternatives are more healthful according to most parameters, but lower sodium was not one of them.[563] The same rough equivalence was found in Brazil.[564] In Australia, plant-based meats were found to have significantly lower sodium content, but that speaks more to the high salt levels in meat,[565] since very few of the meat-free options could be considered low-sodium foods.[566]

In Europe, average sodium levels of conventional versus plant-based meats were similar in Sweden,[567] lower in plant-based meats than conventional in Germany,[568] and higher in France.[569] In the largest single study, which was conducted across five countries in Europe, plant-based meats were found to contain less salt than either red meat or poultry products,[570] but a 2025 systematic review found that the average levels were not significantly different overall. There were, however, some extreme outliers with some plant-based meats exceeding 1,400 milligrams,[571] meaning one serving would take up more than half the maximum of 2,300 milligrams recommended by the U.S. Dietary Guidelines[572] or almost reach the American Heart Association's recommended limit of only 1,500 daily milligrams.[573]

A 2024 systematic review found that while most comparisons were not significantly different, it varied by category. For example, all the plant-based ground meats were higher in sodium, and most of the plant-based processed meats were lower. In fact, the saltiest plant-based sausage was less salty than the least salty meat sausage, but it's the opposite when looking at whole cuts of meat, like steaks or filets.[574]

Researchers did not account for sodium commonly added to meat during preparation, though, which is an issue applicable to nearly every study on this topic.[575] For example, in one study of U.S. products, plant-based burgers had nearly 10 times the sodium as beef, but that's because instead of comparing burgers to burgers, the researchers compared pre-seasoned plant-based burgers to raw beef in an apparent attempt to skew the results.[576]

Similarly, in the French study I mentioned, the substitution of animal-based meat with plant-based meat resulted in an average daily increase in sodium intake from 3,200 milligrams to 3,400 milligrams, but the researchers didn't take into account the fact that people tend to add salt when preparing meat dishes, so there may be little difference in salt levels in the end.[577] This could explain the large discrepancy between plant- versus animal-based ground meat.[578] When comparing apples to apples—for example, conventional meatballs to plant-based meatballs—even the saltiest plant-based meatball is less salty than the least salty meaty meatball.[579]

In terms of burgers, plant-based advocates note the Impossible Whopper "only" contains 10% more sodium than the traditional beef Whopper.[580] Perhaps the reason they just cite a percentage is because both sandwiches have an ungodly 1,000 milligrams or so of sodium each.[581] The salt content of typical non-fast-food meat burgers is usually in the 300 to 700 milligram range,[582] which is in the range of what researchers found people prefer in taste tests,[583] and what is more typically found in plant-based burgers.[584]

Although plant-based meats tend to be higher in fiber and lower in both saturated fat and cholesterol, the fact that they average similar sodium levels as conventional meat may negate some of their advantages for cardiovascular protection.[585] A 2024 systematic review identified 10 studies that looked at the health impact of consuming plant-based meat and concluded that no negative effects had ever been found.[586] But literally the day after the review was accepted, a study out of Singapore was published that called that conclusion into question.[587]

Researchers randomized people to plant-based meats with triple the sodium of the meat that was being replaced, and there was a blunting of the healthy dip in nocturnal diastolic blood pressure normally seen in the early morning hours, which may be attributable to the extra sodium load.[588]

The reliability of nocturnal blood pressure changes is questionable,[589] however, given the poor night-to-night reproducibility.[590] A more accepted predictor of cardiovascular disease risk is daytime diastolic pressure, and that was actually lower in the plant-based group despite the extra sodium. Also, the daytime blood pressure measurement was taken in a clinic and had the benefit of preserved randomization, whereas the nighttime measurements were taken in a nonrandomized subset of volunteers.[591]

The only other randomized controlled trial to rigorously compare the cardiometabolic health effects of plant-based meats with their animal-based counterparts[592] is the Stanford SWAP-MEAT trial, which used products with similar sodium levels to conventional meat and resulted in no difference in blood pressure.[593] Had meat been swapped instead with beans, we would have expected to see a drop in systolic blood pressure, the most important blood pressure predictor of risk,[594] but, in terms of the products they were meant to replace, plant-based meats generally seem to be comparable when it comes to sodium.[595]

Packaging Chemicals and Microplastics

One might expect the amount of leaching of packaging chemicals to be similar between plant- and animal-based products, though the link between poultry consumption and phthalate chemicals in our blood may not be due just to the plastic wrap on meat since eggs have also been implicated.[596] This suggests that the chickens themselves are contaminated at the farm.

In terms of microplastics, both plant- and animal-based products have been found to be similarly contaminated.[597]

Satiety

What about the lack of satiety typical of ultra-processed foods that contributes to overeating?[598] The satiating effect of plant-based meats is one of the best-studied health outcomes. From eight randomized, controlled, cross-over trials of plant-based versus animal-based meat, overall, superior satiety following consumption of plant-based meat was reported, which translated into not only lower caloric intake at that meal, but sometimes even at a following meal hours later.[599] This may be attributed to two factors: the higher fiber content of plant-based products (there is no fiber in meat) and a beneficial modulation of gastrointestinal hormones. For example, the appetite-suppressing satiety hormone GLP-1 mimicked by weight-loss drugs like Ozempic.[600]

In one randomized cross-over trial, researchers tested the effects of two meals matched in calories and macronutrients on GLP-1—a plant-based burger versus a conventional meat burger. Compared to the meat meal, the plant-based meal boosted GLP-1 levels by 40% in both individuals with and without diabetes.[601] The plant-based burger increased satiety more than a calorie- and macronutrient-matched meat burger in all groups of participants tested.[602] But does this actually translate into eating less?

When study participants had a pasta lunch at an all-you-can-eat buffet with either ground plant-based meat or ground beef, they consumed significantly fewer calories of the pasta with the plant-based meat. Yet, despite eating less, they felt just as satisfied, full, and satiated.[603]

Looking at the effects of mycoprotein-based[604] meat substitutes like Quorn, made from the mushroom kingdom rather than the plant kingdom,[605] consumption of mycoprotein results in a decrease in caloric intake at an all-you-can-eat meal and also suppresses subsequent appetite. The effect was enough to significantly decrease intake throughout the subsequent 24-hour period.[606] When researchers compared it to eating chicken, they saw a significantly decreased caloric intake during the mycoprotein meal that was not compensated for later in the day, which led to an average caloric reduction over the whole day by 188 calories.[607]

Mycoprotein-based products may be the healthiest of meats since they are based on a whole food, rather than a protein isolate. They tend to have the most fiber and less sodium and saturated fat compared to other meat substitutes.[608] The only reason certain mycoprotein products are technically ultra-processed is because they contain added ingredients like natural flavors, but the mycoprotein food itself can be considered a whole food that has been used in traditional fermented foods dating back centuries.[609]

Weight Gain

Normally, ultra-processed foods cause people to compulsively eat more and gain weight, but does the increased satiety from plant-based meats translate into eating less and losing weight? In the RE-MAP study, participants were randomized to receive advice to continue their regular diet or replace some of the meat they had been eating with plant-based meat. Although the intervention group swapped out less than a single daily serving of meat, they lost significantly more weight within four weeks.[610]

In the Stanford SWAP-MEAT trial, participants were instructed to replace two or more daily servings of organic and grass-fed beef, pork, and chicken meat with plant-based beef, pork, and chicken while keeping everything else—such as exercise, activity, and sleep—the same for eight weeks. During the plant-based meat phase, they inadvertently lost a couple of pounds. Typically, one would expect weight *gain* after switching from whole foods to ultra-processed products, but when the whole food is meat, switching to plant-based meat caused a modest but significant drop in weight. Notably, this weight loss occurred despite no differences in reported total caloric intake or physical activity levels between the phases.[611]

How can the same calories result in more weight loss? We've seen this before with randomized controlled trials of vegetarian diets. Same caloric restriction, yet more weight loss, a slimmer waist, and less body fat, thanks to eating less meat.[612] That may be due to the fewer branched-chain amino acids in plant-based meat,[613] which would be expected to improve our metabolic health.[614] Or, it may be because the resting metabolic rate in those eating vegetarian[615] is as much as 20% higher, so they're basically burning more calories in their sleep.[616]

Regardless of the mechanism, a significantly lower body weight was reported in two out of three randomized controlled trials in which study participants replaced the meat in some meals with meat alternatives.[617] The slight half-pound drop in weight during the eight weeks in the plant-based group in the third study out of Singapore did not reach statistical significance.[618]

Blood Sugars

How do plant-based meats fare when it comes to endocrine disorders, namely type 2 diabetes?

A 2024 systematic review of population studies on the association of different protein sources and the risk of developing diabetes found that a significant and dose-dependent increase in the risk of type 2 diabetes is linked with long-term consumption of protein from animals, but not protein from plants. In fact, researchers found that diabetes risk may fall by 20% with every 20 grams of animal protein replaced with plant protein. But the plant protein they're talking about is mostly from whole, minimally processed, or traditionally processed plant foods, like legumes, grains, and nuts.[619]

The same was seen with most interventional trials. Randomized controlled studies found that replacing sources of animal protein with plant protein improves both short-term and long-term blood sugar control in people with diabetes. Again, though, in most cases, the plant proteins replacing the animal proteins were from whole plant foods, like beans or nuts.[620] Ultra-processed foods tend to be associated with worsening blood sugar control,[621] but might plant-based meats be the ultra-processed exception here, too?

Individuals with diabetes were randomized to replace half their animal protein intake with an ultra-processed soy product called TVP (textured vegetable protein) for four years. It remains the longest interventional trial ever published on plant-based meat. Compared to those in the control group, blood sugar control significantly improved in those who replaced half their animal protein with TVP.[622]

Replacing even a single daily serving of red meat with TVP for eight weeks can lead to a significant improvement in insulin resistance, the cause of type 2 diabetes, though only a whole soy food was able to additionally improve fasting blood sugars significantly within that same period.[623] In one of the most extraordinary studies, pregnant women with gestational diabetes replacing half the animal protein in their diet with plant-based TVP not only led to a significant improvement in their blood sugar control and insulin resistance, but the number of newborn hospitalizations was slashed by 85%.[624]

TVP is unusual, though, in that it has zero saturated fat and zero sodium. In the Stanford SWAP-MEAT study that used Beyond Meat products, researchers found no significant difference in participants' insulin or blood sugar levels,[625] and the same was seen in the Singapore study that also used more conventional plant-based meats. There were no differences in day-to-day blood sugar control, week-to-week control, or insulin resistance. In a nonrandomized subset with continuous glucose monitoring, one measure even appeared better in the conventional meat group, but the other 18 measures did not.[626]

An observational study found that consumers of Quorn appeared to have better short- and long-term blood sugar control after controlling for a long list of factors, but causal conclusions cannot be drawn from a snapshot-in-time study.[627] When put to the test, researchers found that participants' insulin levels were lower immediately after a meal while achieving the same blood sugar control.[628] This suggested that mycoprotein may improve insulin sensitivity,[629] and, indeed, when formally tested, mycoprotein-based chicken resulted in a significant improvement in insulin sensitivity compared to chicken using multiple measures in adults[630] who were as overweight as average Americans.[631] However, daily Quorn consumption doesn't appear to affect insulin sensitivity among those classified as ideal weight.[632]

Overall, depending on the types of plant-based meat and population, most studies find that plant-based meats are about the same or better when it comes to blood sugar control.[633]

Gut Microbiome

Do plant-based meats harm the gut microbiome as other ultra-processed foods have been suspected of doing? Apparently not: All three interventional studies addressing the question showed that plant-based meats offered at least some microbiome benefits compared to conventional meat.

In a study titled "The Impact of Plant-Based Meat Alternatives on the Gut Microbiota of Consumers: A Real-World Study," researchers conducted a randomized controlled trial to assess changes to the gut microbiome by analyzing stool samples before and after study participants replaced five meals of meat a week with plant-based meat. One of the greatest challenges in defining a good gut microbiome is that we are still in the early stages of understanding its complexity. However, one of the "indisputable criteria" for a healthy gut is a plethora of fiber feeders that turn the fiber we eat into anti-inflammatory compounds, and that's exactly what the researchers found.

Even though the fiber content of ultra-processed plant-based meats pales in comparison to whole plant foods like beans, when the study participants replaced conventional meat with plant-based meat, about 20 grams of fiber were added to their weekly diet. The researchers concluded that even just the "occasional replacement of animal meats with PBMA [plant-based meat alternatives]...may promote positive changes to the gut microbiome of consumers."[634]

In the second trial, the Mycomeat study, participants were randomized to replace a few daily servings of meat for two weeks with the mycoprotein-based meat Quorn. The title says it all: "Substituting Meat for Mycoprotein Reduces Genotoxicity and Increases the Abundance of Beneficial Microbes in the Gut." Fecal genotoxicity is the amount of DNA damage that feces cause to colon cells. The lower genotoxicity may be due to the participants cutting down on meat, but on the mycoprotein, there was a boost in good gut bacteria, like *Lactobacillus*, which may protect against cancer, at least in rodent models. This suggests that the fiber in mycoprotein products may have beneficial prebiotic potential.[635]

The two-week swap did not seem to be a long enough duration to affect TMAO levels,[636] but, in the eight-week SWAP-MEAT study, replacing two or more daily servings of beef, pork, and chicken with plant-based beef, pork, and chicken improved several cardiovascular disease risk factors, including TMAO, trimethylamine-n-oxide.[637]

TMAO is considered to be a smoking gun in gut microbiome-disease interactions.[638] When we eat meat, dairy, or eggs, certain bad gut bugs turn the carnitine and choline into trimethylamine, which is oxidized by our liver into TMAO, and that appears to cause havoc within our body.[639] So, the cardiovascular harm from consuming eggs and meat may come from more than just their cholesterol and saturated fat.[640]

TMAO is linked to nearly every one of our leading causes of death: cardiovascular disease (killer number one), cancer (number two), stroke (number four),[641] chronic lung disease (number five),[642] Alzheimer's disease (number six),[643] diabetes (number seven),[644] kidney disease (number eight),[645] liver disease (number nine),[646] hypertension (number 13),[647] and Parkinson's disease (killer number 15).[648]

The probability values, commonly known as *P values*, linking TMAO to these killer diseases reached 10^{-22}. *P values* are used as a measure of the strength of evidence. A *P value* like 10^{-22} means we would only get a connection between TMAO and disease that extreme by chance if the study was run about a billion trillion times. So, as the title of a metabolic diseases journal commentary suggested, maybe TMAO should also stand for "Time to Minimize Intake of Animal Products."[649] We can do that by switching to plant products.

The Acid Test

Plant-based meals can also be better for our *upper* digestive tract. When study participants were randomized to eat chicken, cheese, fish, and steak versus tofu, soy steaks, seitan, and veggie burgers, they experienced twice as many acid reflux symptoms like heartburn after the animal-protein meal than the plant-protein meal. When researchers stuck a probe down their throats, they discovered that, after consuming the animal products, the participants had three times as much acid refluxing up from their stomach into their esophagus.[650]

Inflammation and Artery Function

In the SWAP-MEAT study, there were several improvements in cardiovascular disease risk factors, but no changes were seen in markers of inflammation. The authors suggest the eight-week study may have been too short to achieve detectable improvements in systemic inflammation,[651] but a healthy enough diet without any meat can cut inflammatory markers, like C-reactive protein and IL-6, by as much as 30% in half the time, within four weeks.[652]

The lack of changes in inflammation markers may instead have been because the study used Beyond Meat products, which at the time contained coconut oil. Although the participants were consuming less saturated fat than those in the meat group, the level may still have been too high.[653] Saturated fat is the single most pro-inflammatory food component in the dietary inflammatory index.[654] After consuming just one Sausage and Egg McMuffin meal, for example, inflammatory markers can double within four hours.[655]

What if meat were replaced with a healthier plant-based meat like TVP, which has almost no fat? C-reactive protein levels, that common marker of systemic inflammation, can drop by 75%.[656] Replacing one serving of meat a day for eight weeks with a whole soy food worked even better, and for markers of artery function, only the whole soy food seemed to help.[657] Even a single day of plant-based meals has been shown to improve markers of artery function, but the study included some less-processed plant foods like tofu.[658]

Instead of measuring *markers* of arterial function, what about measuring *actual* arterial function after replacing 25 daily grams of animal protein with soy protein? Study participants had a significant improvement in their arterial function that disappeared when they went back to consuming animal protein.[659] Two percent of the soy was in the form of tofu, but the other 98% was in the form of ultra-processed soy-based meat and dairy products.[660]

Oxidative Stress

What about oxidative stress, excessive free radical damage that may be caused by run-of-the-mill ultra-processed foods? Swapping half of one's animal protein intake with TVP not only improved blood sugar control and insulin resistance, but it also reduced levels of MDA,[661] which is the most commonly used biomarker for oxidative stress.[662]

Replacing just one daily serving of red meat with TVP led to a significant drop in oxidative stress and a significant boost in the total antioxidant capacity of the participants' bloodstream within eight weeks.[663] This makes sense, since the antioxidant content of even ultra-processed plant-based burgers averages twice that of beef burgers.[664] After a single meal of a conventional meat burger versus a veggie burger, researchers found that only the plant-based one ameliorated oxidative stress, indicating the therapeutic potential of plant-based nutrition—even in the form of an ultra-processed product—to provide "better protection against the development of complications associated with diabetes and obesity."[665]

The Ultra-Processed Exception

In summary, Figure 9 shows how conventional meat compares to ultra-processed plant-based meat, including all the factors suggested by the developer of the NOVA system to explain why typical ultra-processed foods may contribute to morbidity and mortality.[666]

Normally, when ultra-processed products are compared to the foods they were intended to replace—Lucky Charms versus oatmeal or fruit-flavored candy versus fruit—the designer foods don't just have a junkier nutrient profile; they are inferior across a wide array of metrics. But when meat is supplanted by plants—even ultra-processed ones—plant-based meats appear to be the exception in that they are *better* in most ways compared to the foods they were designed to replace.

As you can see in Figure 9, plant-based meat tends to score nutritionally healthier than meat, based on every study using every major nutrient profiling system. They also tend to have fewer calories per serving and are no worse than conventional meat when it comes to texture or matrix degradation. Plant-based meat also has more healthful phytonutrients, fewer or similar levels of toxic AGEs (depending on detection method), no worse levels of the heat-induced contaminants furosine and acrylamide, and fewer carcinogenic heterocyclic amines and polycyclic aromatic hydrocarbons.

Conventional Meat vs. Ultra-Processed Plant-Based Meat

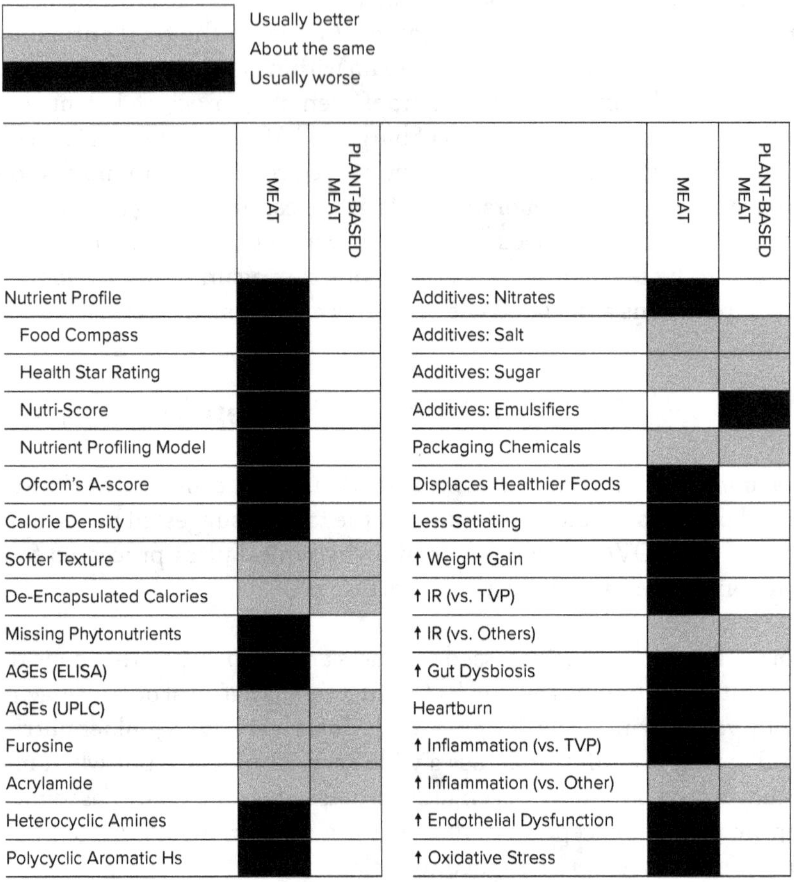

Legend:
- ☐ Usually better (white)
- ▒ About the same (gray)
- ■ Usually worse (black)

	MEAT	PLANT-BASED MEAT		MEAT	PLANT-BASED MEAT
Nutrient Profile	■	☐	Additives: Nitrates	■	☐
Food Compass	■	☐	Additives: Salt	▒	▒
Health Star Rating	■	☐	Additives: Sugar	▒	▒
Nutri-Score	■	☐	Additives: Emulsifiers	☐	■
Nutrient Profiling Model	■	☐	Packaging Chemicals	▒	▒
Ofcom's A-score	■	☐	Displaces Healthier Foods	■	☐
Calorie Density	■	☐	Less Satiating	■	☐
Softer Texture	▒	▒	↑ Weight Gain	■	☐
De-Encapsulated Calories	▒	▒	↑ IR (vs. TVP)	■	☐
Missing Phytonutrients	■	☐	↑ IR (vs. Others)	▒	▒
AGEs (ELISA)	■	☐	↑ Gut Dysbiosis	■	☐
AGEs (UPLC)	▒	▒	Heartburn	■	☐
Furosine	▒	▒	↑ Inflammation (vs. TVP)	■	☐
Acrylamide	▒	▒	↑ Inflammation (vs. Other)	▒	▒
Heterocyclic Amines	■	☐	↑ Endothelial Dysfunction	■	☐
Polycyclic Aromatic Hs	■	☐	↑ Oxidative Stress	■	☐

Figure 9

Plant-based meat tends to be better when it comes to some additives, like carcinogenic nitrite preservatives, similar with salt and sugar, and worse with emulsifiers. Leached chemicals from packaging should be similar. Plant-based meat is also more satiating, causes less weight gain, and is either better than or no different when it comes to insulin resistance (depending on the type of product). Plant-based meat is also superior when it comes to our gut health, including our microbiome, heartburn symptoms, and acid reflux; better or no different when it comes to inflammation (depending on the type of product); and probably superior when it comes to arterial function and oxidative stress.[667]

The bottom line is that unlike almost any other ultra-processed products, plant-based meats appear to be the rare case in which ultra-processed products are better, overall, than the foods they were designed to replace. Now, this probably says less about how healthy they are and more about the unhealthfulness of modern meat. Take, for example, food safety.

FOOD SAFETY

A lobbying group funded by the tobacco, alcohol, and meat industries aired a television ad during the Super Bowl[668] that questioned plant-based meat for its hard-to-spell ingredients like *methylcellulose*.[669] Impossible Foods responded with a spelling bee parody of its own, questioning an unintentional additive in conventional meat: *poop*.[670]

Foodborne Fecal Bacteria

Fecal contamination of the carcass in the slaughter plant is considered unavoidable.[671] Although methods exist to remove visible contamination of feces from meat[672] and there are experimental imaging technologies designed to detect more "diluted fecal contaminations,"[673] we're still left at the retail level with widespread contamination with fecal bacteria. *Enterococci* are used as markers of fecal contamination of food products. It was found in 85% of ground beef and turkey, about 50% of chicken, and about a third of pork sampled nationally by the U.S. Department of Agriculture.[674]

But you don't have to cook the crap out of plant-based meat, because there shouldn't be any crap to begin with.

Fecal contamination of foods isn't just unsavory, but a critical public health issue.[675] Fecal matter is considered the main source of some of our most serious foodborne pathogens, including *Salmonella* and *Campylobacter*.[676] *Salmonella* is the leading cause of foodborne-related hospitalization and death.[677] One in four packages of retail chicken sampled in the United States is contaminated with the pathogen, one in eight samples of ground turkey, one in 24 packages of pork, and one in 67 packages of ground beef.[678]

Campylobacter, which sickens more than 800,000 Americans a year,[679] is also found in every three or four packages of retail chicken.[680] Simply shopping for meat can be risky, as disease-causing fecal bacteria can contaminate the outer packaging of meat.[681]

"While these statistics seem discouraging," a review in *Microbial Physiology* concluded, "food-borne illnesses are largely preventable, and the simplest approach to reduce their occurrences is to greatly reduce the consumption of meat, dairy, fish, and poultry."[682] They're caused by intestinal bugs; plants don't have intestines, so we can reduce our risk with plant-based meat. Although there have been cases of manure run-off contaminating crops, poultry is the leading cause of outbreaks of food poisoning, followed by fish, then beef.[683]

The top five pathogen–food combinations that cause the greatest burden of disease in terms of years of healthy life lost are: (1) *Campylobacter* in poultry, (2) *Toxoplasma* in pork, (3) *Listeria* in deli meats, (4) *Salmonella* in poultry, and (5) *Listeria* in dairy.[684]

Viruses, Prions, and Parasites

Toxoplasma is a brain parasite that may infect a million Americans every year, making it a leading cause of severe foodborne illness in the United States.[685] What may end up in our brain may start in our burger.[686]

Tapeworms in the human brain from pork consumption have also become an increasingly important emerging infection in the United States.[687] What you think is a migraine may not be a migraine.[688] That is what was reportedly found in the brain of the reigning U.S. Secretary of Health and Human Services.

Shockingly, nearly half a million urinary tract infections may be blamed on *E. coli*-infected meat, particularly poultry.[689] We can get viral hepatitis (hepatitis E) from pork.[690] Plants don't make prions, either, the causes of fatal spongiform brain diseases.[691] There's a reason there's a mad cow disease but not a mad Quorn disease.

Antibiotic Residues and Resistance

To compensate for overcrowded, stressful, unhygienic conditions in typical intensive farming systems, animals raised for food are dosed *en masse*[692] with 10 million pounds of medically important antibiotics each year. In the United States alone, farm animals are given more than a million pounds of penicillin drugs and 4,000 tons of tetracyclines. Antibiotics important to human medicine are laced into the feed and water of cows, pigs, chickens, and fish by the thousands of tons annually.[693]

Such agricultural applications for antimicrobials are considered an "urgent threat to human health," with the link between the use of antibiotics in animals raised for food and the antibiotic resistance in humans considered "unequivocal."[694] This contributes to the millions of antibiotic-resistant infections Americans suffer every year and the tens of thousands of deaths, according to the Centers for Disease Control and Prevention.[695]

Most of the *Salmonella* and *Campylobacter* in chicken breasts sold in U.S. stores have been found to be resistant to at least one class of antibiotics, and about half the *Salmonella* was resistant to three or more classes of drugs.[696] Eating meat contaminated with antibiotic-resistant bacteria is considered a "severe health hazard."[697]

Even organic meat from animals raised without antibiotics may be contaminated with multidrug-resistant bacteria, perhaps through cross-contamination at slaughter.[698] In a cover story, *Consumer Reports* urged retailers to stop selling meat produced with antibiotics and noted some store "employee confusion": "An assistant manager at one grocery store, when asked by a shopper for meats raised without antibiotics, responded, 'Wait, you mean like veggie burgers?'"[699]

Maybe they aren't so confused after all.

Antibiotic-resistance genes[700] can also be transmitted through meat, before transferring to other pathogens in our gut.[701] Residues of the antibiotic drugs themselves can, too, which is considered another serious public health threat.[702] In fact, how much meat we eat correlates to the trace levels of antibiotics we pee out every day.[703] These drug residues may cause allergies, nerve damage, liver damage, reproductive disorders, and bone marrow toxicity. They may also increase cancer risk.[704] And just imagine what eating antibiotics every day could be doing to disrupt our gut microbiome.[705] In contrast, the production of plant-based meats involves no guts, no feces, and no antibiotics.

Comparing Microbial Loads

This is not to say that plant-based meats are sterile.[706] They can become contaminated with spoilage bacteria like any other food. That's why they are typically sold frozen or refrigerated.[707] They can still foster the growth of bacteria but start out with lower indigenous microbial loads. Ground beef, for example, starts out with a hundred times more bacterial contamination than what has been found in Impossible Burgers and Beyond Burgers.[708]

Any food, once made, can become contaminated, but plant-based meats start out with bacterial levels[709] that are a thousand times lower than the relatively stringent limits for ground beef in the U.S. National School Lunch Program.[710] And, of course, the *types* of bacteria are what matter.[711] The primary causes of food poisoning are *E. coli*, *Salmonella*, and *Campylobacter*, and plant-based meats shouldn't start out with any of these poo-based bacteria.[712] Most bacteria found in plant-based meats are lactic acid bacteria. There are spore-forming bacteria that may survive the production process, though, so plant-based meats need to be kept refrigerated.[713]

OTHER HEALTH CONSIDERATIONS

Antibiotics aren't the only drugs with which farm animals are dosed that have potential public health implications.

Hormones

Currently, seven hormone drugs are approved by the FDA to bulk up U.S. production of milk and meat.[714] In Europe, there exists a total ban on such use out of an abundance of caution due to potential cancer risk. However, even without injected or implanted hormones, animal products naturally contain hormones because the meat, eggs, and milk come from animals.[715] Cow's milk can as much as quadruple the estrogen levels of men and prepubescent children within hours of consumption.[716]

In contrast, there are hormone-like molecules called *phytohormones* in plants, like genistein, the soy phytoestrogen,[717] which appears to have a variety of health benefits. These include antioxidant, anti-inflammatory, anti-diabetes, and anti-cancer effects.[718] For example, genistein appears to reduce the risk of breast cancer,[719] while animal estrogens increase it.[720,721] Genistein may also improve breast cancer survival.[722] Soy phytoestrogens share some of the benefits of human hormones, like preserving our bone mass[723] and decreasing menopausal symptoms,[724] apparently without disrupting thyroid function or our reproductive health[725] or adversely affecting male hormones like testosterone.[726]

Industrial Pollutants

I've discussed processing contaminants, but there are also *industrial* pollutants that build up in the food chain into meat, such as certain pesticides, PCBs, heavy metals, and flame retardant chemicals.[727]

Can't we just buy organic meat? Surprisingly, sticking to organic meat does not seem to diminish the carcinogenic potential of meat-borne industrial pollutants.[728] In a study looking at the micropollutants and chemical residues in organic versus conventional meats, several environmental contaminants—including dioxins, PCBs, lead, and arsenic—were measured at significantly higher levels in organic samples.[729] Cooking can help draw off some of the fat where PCBs are concentrated,[730] but, in seafood, cooking generally increases the concentration of contaminants like mercury.[731] Plant-based tuna, however, is mercury-free.[732]

When researchers tested retail meat for the presence of 33 chemicals with calculated carcinogenic potential, such as organochlorine pesticides like DDT and dioxin-like PCBs,[733] they concluded that, in order to reduce the risk of cancer, ingestion of beef, pork, or chicken should be limited to a maximum of five servings a *month*.[734]

Other Potential Cancer Contributors

When the International Agency for Research on Cancer classified processed meat as a known human carcinogen and unprocessed meat as a probable human carcinogen,[735] it was not because of carcinogenic environmental pollutants.[736] Rather, the classifications focused on the N-nitroso compounds formed in meat, as well as the two classes of cooked meat carcinogens, heterocyclic amines and polycyclic aromatic hydrocarbons.

Those are considered among the primary mechanisms by which meat can cause colorectal cancer.[737] Less likely candidates found in meat that have been hypothesized to contribute to cancer risk include arachidonic acid, excess methionine or sulfur-containing amino acids in general, trans fats, the effects of animal protein on the human hormone IGF-1, formaldehyde, carcinogenic viruses, saturated fats, Neu5Gc, TMAO,[738] and other uremic toxins produced through putrefaction in the colon.[739] How do these putative mechanisms compare between meat made from animals versus plants?

Arachidonic Acid

Arachidonic acid is a pro-inflammatory, long-chain omega-6 fat,[740] and meat, including chicken, beef, pork, and fish, is our main dietary source.[741] When directly compared, beef had greater quantities of arachidonic acid than plant-based meat.[742]

Methionine

I dedicated an entire chapter on methionine restriction in my longevity book *How Not to Age*. Like sodium, methionine is an essential nutrient, but we can get too much. There is mounting evidence that concentrations of certain amino acids, including methionine, which are higher in animal protein than plant protein, may exert adverse effects on our metabolism.[743] Methionine restriction is considered a feasible strategy for lifespan extension[744] and fighting against age-related disease.[745] It can also be exploited for treating cancer.[746]

Methionine has been found to be 20-fold lower in plant-based burgers[747] and shown to successfully lower levels in consumers' bloodstream.[748]

Trans Fats

Beef burgers naturally contain twice as many trans fats as plant-based burgers.[749]

IGF-1

IGF-1 is a growth hormone that appears to be causally associated with multiple cancers, including those of the breast[750] and prostate.[751] Lower blood levels of IGF-1 among those eating plant-based[752] may help explain why vegans have up to 39% lower overall risk of developing cancer, compared to the general public.[753]

Replacing all animal protein in the diet with plant protein can significantly lower IGF-1 levels within four weeks,[754] but swapping out only a few daily servings of conventional meat for plant-based meat appears insufficient to significantly lower levels of this cancer-promoting hormone.[755]

Formaldehyde

Formaldehyde can be formed in meat from the breakdown of muscle or the stress hormone adrenaline, but it can also be formed in other ways.[756] For instance, heated soy protein isolate, a component of many plant-based meats, can reach levels as high as 2.7 milligrams per kilogram,[757] but the amount found naturally in meat tends to be higher, though the amounts in both are negligible.[758] The tolerable upper daily limit for formaldehyde is about 20 milligrams a day, which could allow for around 10 meat burgers or 300 veggie burgers a day.[759]

Carcinogenic Viruses

There are reasons to suspect the involvement of bovine viruses in colorectal cancer.[760] So-called *hamburger polyomaviruses* can survive typical meat cooking temperatures.[761] A specific class of infectious agents has been isolated from both cows and areas around human colon cancer tissue[762] (as well as in the brains of people with multiple sclerosis).[763] Shockingly, some researchers have estimated that as many as 37% of breast cancer cases may be attributable to exposure to bovine leukemia virus,[764] presumably through consumption of meat and/or dairy.[765] All of these infectious agents would presumably be absent in plant-based meat.

Saturated Fats and Sulfur-Containing Amino Acids

Less speculatively, cancer may be driven by the oxidative stress and inflammation triggered by interactions between saturated fats or sulfur-containing amino acids and our gut microbiome.[766] Rats receiving fecal transplants from animals fed meat developed more precancerous lesions in their colons, demonstrating the pro-cancer influence of meat on the gut microbiome, at least in rodents.[767] In humans, there appear to be microbial signatures specific to colorectal cancer,[768] including cancer-related bacteria such as *Bilophila wadsworthia*,[769] whose growth is facilitated by saturated fat[770] and the sulfur-containing amino acids concentrated in animal products.[771]

About four dozen studies have compared saturated fat levels in plant-based meats versus comparable meat products, and about 25% found no significant differences in levels, while the other 75% found significantly lower levels in the plant-based options.[772] Upon reviewing the saturated fat content of more than 500 plant-based meats, every category was found to average significantly lower than regular meat, though there are some extreme outliers.[773] Plant-based meats also tend to be lower in sulfur-containing amino acids, with the exception of one product from China that contained cheese.[774]

Neu5Gc

Neu5Gc is a sialic acid that is not made by plants. The problem is that it isn't made by humans either, so when we incorporate it into our body by eating meat from animals that do make it, our immune system treats it as a foreign invader, triggering an immune response.[775] We produce antibodies to attack Neu5Gc lodged in our tissues, which causes an autoimmune process, leading to inflammation that appears to facilitate the survival and spread of cancer cells.[776]

TMAO

There may also be a strong link between colorectal cancer and the meat metabolite TMAO mentioned previously.[777] As noted, the Stanford SWAP-MEAT study found that we can get a significant drop in TMAO levels by replacing a few daily servings of organic meat with plant-based meat.[778]

Putrefaction Products

Maybe part of the increased cancer risk is from meat putrefying in our colon. Putrefaction involves the decomposition of undigested proteins in the gut, some of the by-products of which have been implicated in the development of colorectal cancer.[779] But can't plant proteins putrefy, too? There have been studies of plant-based meat swaps for two such putrefaction products, ammonia and cresol, a uremic toxin that appears to promote the invasion and migration of cancer cells.[780] They both found beneficial impacts.

The first randomized clinical trial found that a plant-based burger with the same amount of protein as a conventional meat burger generated significantly less ammonia. Ammonia buildup can be a serious problem in liver cirrhosis.[781] The other trial found that replacing a few daily servings of steak, sausages, ham, bacon, ground beef, and hot dogs with the same amount of protein in the form of meat-free Quorn steak, sausages, ham, bacon, ground beef, and hot dogs for two weeks led to a significant drop in cresol exposure.[782]

Mold Toxins

The only contaminants I could find at potentially higher levels in plant-based meat are certain agricultural mold toxins, which are practically unavoidable, as they affect about a quarter of the world's crops.[783] Although moldy feed crops can lead to contaminated animal products, the levels in meat are generally lower than in plants. More than 100 samples of plant-based meat have been tested—all from Europe—and the levels are such that, if everyone switched to 100% plant-based meat, intake of a few contaminants, like the liver carcinogen aflatoxin, would exceed safety levels and present a potential food safety risk.[784]

The first published risk analysis acknowledged that shifting to plant-based meat would eliminate the colorectal cancer risk from animal meat; however, if these mold toxins are not regulated, we could end up with more cases of liver cancer.[785] Researchers estimated that the potential risk of liver cancer for those who exclusively ate plant-based meat would be low, affecting up to one individual out of every two million people who made the switch.[786] So, although there would be less cancer overall, plant-based meat companies should be screening their raw ingredients. The problem of moldy crops is only expected to worsen in the context of our changing climate.[787]

Allergens

All in all, plant-based meat is better than conventional meat in at least 30 different ways, but aside from the emulsifiers and mold toxins, the only other potential downside of meat from plants rather than animals would be certain food allergies. Although the majority of dietary allergies are to animal products,[788] allergies to land-based meat are rare—that is, unless you've been bitten by certain types of ticks. (If you're unfamiliar with that fascinating story, check out my video on the subject at see.nf/tick.)

There have been rare, authenticated reports of people with Quorn allergies[789] and even more with unvalidated complaints.[790] However, given how many packages of Quorn have been sold, the rate of allergic reactions may be on the order of around one in nine million.[791] There haven't been any confirmed cases of allergy to the mycoprotein used in other brands such as The Better Meat Co.[792]

About 1 in 150 people are allergic to wheat or soy,[793] though, which can be common components in plant-based meats.

Dietary Acid Load

Dietary acid load is determined by the balance of foods that induce the formation of acid in the body, like meat and eggs, against alkaline-forming foods, like fruits and vegetables.[794] Diets with a high acid load can induce a low-grade metabolic acidosis, which is associated with the development of a variety of diseases[795] that affect multiple organ systems[796]—increasing the risk of chronic kidney disease, for example.[797] An acid-generating diet is also associated with an increased risk of cancer,[798] including breast and colon cancers.[799]

The most acid-forming foods are meats, with white meat worse than red,[800] and the most *alkaline*-forming foods are vegetables.[801]

What about plant-based meats? As you can see in Figure 10, the majority exerted a lower acid load compared to their meat-based counterparts. The dashed line on the left indicates the acid load of beef, and the dashed line on the right is where chicken lands.[802]

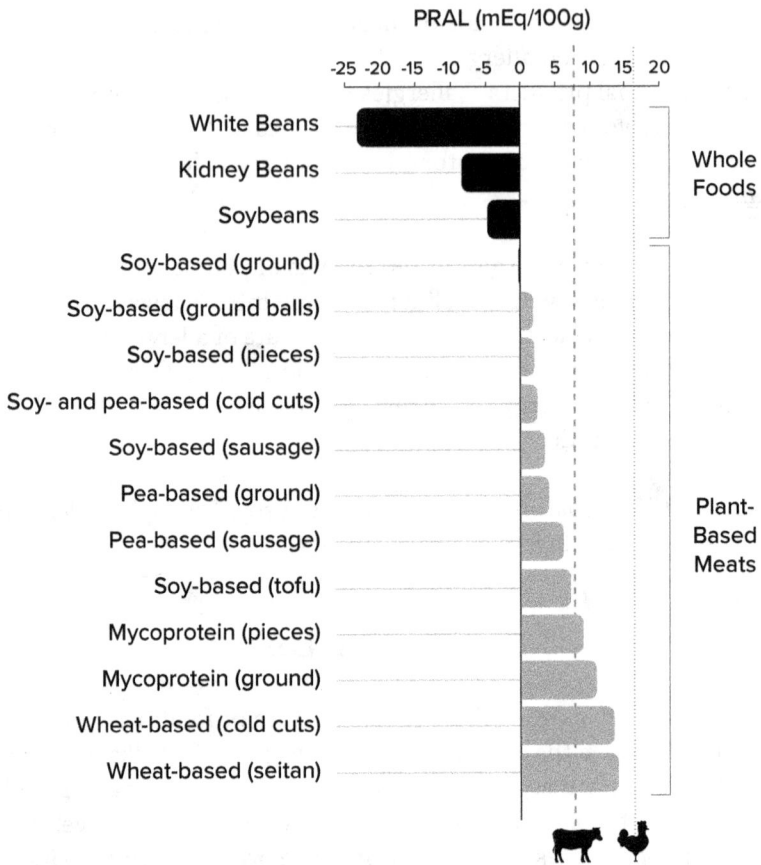

Acid Load of Plant-Based Meats and Beans Compared to Beef and Chicken

PRAL (mEq/100g)

Figure 10

You'll note that while most of the plant- and mycoprotein-based meats do better than conventional meats, they are no match for unprocessed plant foods like beans, which have a negative acid load, meaning they're actively alkaline- or base-forming. The researchers concluded that, although most of the meat-free alternatives were better and "could offer a steppingstone in the transition away from meat to increased plant consumption, they might be unsuitable to substantially alkalize an individual's diet."[803]

We may need beans to really turn up the base, but the Stanford SWAP-MEAT trial did find a small alkalizing effect when it tracked the pH of participants' urine as they swapped out a few daily servings of meat for plant-based meat.[804]

Kidney Function

The SWAP-MEAT study only enrolled healthy adults, so its urinary findings can't tell us if daily plant-based meat consumption would help improve the function of ailing kidneys.[805] But there have been studies of kidney patients. Within eight weeks, a 100% swap of animal protein for the textured soy protein TVP led to a significant improvement in kidney function. In addition to a massive 68-point drop in LDL cholesterol, the study participants experienced a 30% improvement in the amount of protein leaking into their urine. Once they switched back to animal protein, however, their kidneys resumed their decline.[806]

What if we only replaced half our animal protein?

In perhaps the most remarkable study of the effects of partially switching meat for an ultra-processed plant-based alternative, diabetics with failing kidneys were randomized to replace half their animal protein with TVP for four years. (Interventional trials lasting that long in the field of nutrition are lamentably quite rare.) The kidney function of those in the control group continued to get worse over time, but, in the TVP group, their kidney function got *better* year after year. As a bonus, their blood sugar control improved, too, as did their cholesterol and triglycerides. Replacing half their animal protein with ultra-processed plant protein also led to a significant reduction in C-reactive protein levels. That is a sign of decreasing inflammation in the body, which the researchers suggest may be responsible for the reversal of the kidney failure trajectory.[807]

Replacing 50% of study participants' animal protein for more common meat substitutes like veggie burgers was unable to move the needle within eight weeks in patients with diabetic kidney disease,[808] but replacing 50% of their animal protein with TVP resulted in kidney function improving significantly within seven weeks. The kidneys of nearly every patient worsened on the conventional diet in which 70% of their protein came from animal sources, but the kidneys of nearly every individual got better after switching just half their animal protein with plant-based TVP.[809]

What About Nutrient Sufficiency?

I've concentrated on dietary components we're getting too much of—saturated fat, trans fat, cholesterol, salt, and sugar—because, these days, most of us are dying from diseases of excess, not deficiency. Does it matter that plant-based meat has more vitamin C or less riboflavin? How many of us suffer from scurvy or ariboflavinosis?[810] In contrast, how many suffer from diseases of excess saturated fat, salt, sugar, and calories—conditions like heart disease, high blood pressure, stroke, diabetes, obesity, fatty liver, and so on?

But, if one were going to compare nutrient content, the place to start would be where there's an epidemic of deficient intake. Of all the 50 or so vitamins, minerals, and other nutrients tracked in the American diet, the single greatest deficiency is fiber.[811] Only 6% of Americans reach what is considered the "adequate daily intake," which means that 94% of Americans eat fiber-deficient diets.[812] Not surprisingly, plant-based meats have more fiber than any type of conventional meat, which averages zero,[813] as fiber, by definition, is only found in plants.[814]

So, when a comparison study finds that all plant-based meats have more fiber, but some have less protein than their meat counterparts, what should be the takeaway? First, when all the studies are put together, bean-, pea-, and mycoprotein-based plant-based meats typically match conventional meat in protein content.[815] More importantly, though, we are not in the midst of a protein deficiency epidemic, as much as marketing departments try to tell us otherwise.

Protein intakes in high- and middle-income countries tend to far exceed recommended levels.[816] Whereas only 6% of Americans get enough fiber, it's reversed for protein: Only 7% do *not* get enough protein. More than 90% of Americans get enough protein, but more than 90% fail to get enough fiber.[817] Even vegans, who don't eat any meat, eggs, or dairy, tend to get nearly twice[818] the estimated average protein requirement.[819]

Protein claims on packages are more about generating wealth than health. It's like boasting there's 10 times more niacin in meat, but when's the last time you heard of anyone suffering from pellagra?[820] Or bragging about plant-based meat having 500 times more thiamin, but when's the last time you heard of someone with the deficiency disease beriberi?[821]

Less than a quarter of plant-based meats may be fortified with vitamin B12, which could be a problem for vegans,[822] but they aren't the target audience of meat substitutes. The point is to replace some meat with something healthier.[823] Inadequate B12 intake is relatively rare among the general population.[824] For example, doubling the consumption of plant-based meat and reducing the intake of conventional meat by half might lower B12 intake from 170% higher than the RDA of 2.4 down to 140% higher.[825]

What about iron? Few in the overall population fail to get enough iron, but about one in five menstruating women don't consume enough iron to replace losses.[826] A systematic review found that plant-based meats were consistently reported to contain more iron, but what about iron *bioavailability*?[827] That was put to the test using human intestinal cells to see how much iron would be absorbed from soy burgers versus beef burgers, and researchers found that iron bioavailability was comparable between the two. So, if anything, the plant-based burger may end up providing more bioaccessible iron.[828]

Another nutrient of particular concern to reproductive-age women is folate, due to birth defect risk associated with insufficiency.[829] There have been four studies comparing folate levels in plant-based meat versus meat comparators, and they all found that plant-based meat contained in the range of 2 to 28 times more.[830,831,832,833]

HEALTH CONSEQUENCES
OF PLANT-BASED MEAT

Figure 11 synthesizes where we stand on the comparison of ultra-processed plant-based meat to what it's meant to replace. This includes consideration of both the negatives inherent to most ultra-processed products, for which plant-based meats are largely exceptions, and the liabilities typical of meat, which plant-based meats largely alleviate.

Some of these factors are obviously more important than others. For example, the fact that a food like bacon has been officially designated as cancer-causing in humans is more important than the fact it may have a few more calories than plant-based bacon. Meat represents the only scenario in which ultra-processed products were designed to replace foods that we know cause cancer. Many meats we eat are known or probable human carcinogens. These are foods in desperate need of replacement.

But cancer is only killer number two.

Heart Disease Risk Reduction

Killer number one for both men and women is heart disease. Under the nutrient profile in Figure 11 are the three main dietary components that raise LDL (bad) cholesterol: saturated fat, trans fat, and dietary cholesterol. There are certainly other factors that affect heart disease risk, such

Conventional Meat vs.
Ultra-Processed Plant-Based Meat

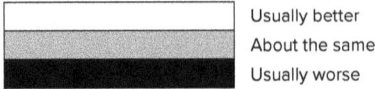

	Usually better
	About the same
	Usually worse

	MEAT	PLANT-BASED MEAT		MEAT	PLANT-BASED MEAT
Nutrient Profile	■		↑ IR (vs. TVP)	■	
Saturated Fat	■		↑ IR (vs. Others)	▨	▨
Trans Fat	■		Heartburn	■	
Cholesterol	■		↑ Gut Dysbiosis	■	
Fiber	■		↑ Inflammation (vs. TVP)	■	
Calorie Density	■		↑ Inflammation (vs. Other)	▨	▨
Softer Texture	▨	▨	↑ Endothelial Dysfunction	■	
De-Encapsulated Calories	▨	▨	↑ Oxidative Stress	■	
Phytonutrients	■		*Salmonella*	■	
Antioxidants	■		*Campylobacter*	■	
AGEs (ELISA)	■		Toxoplasma	■	
AGEs (UPLC)	▨	▨	Antibiotic Resistance	■	
Furosine	▨	▨	Antibiotic Residues	■	
Acrylamide	▨	▨	Hormones	■	
HCAs	■		Pollutants	■	
PAHs	■		Mold Toxins		■
Nitrates	■		Food Allergens		■
Salt	▨	▨	Carcinogen Status	■	
Sugar	▨		Neu5gc	■	
Emulsifiers		■	↑ IGF-1	▨	▨
Packaging Chemicals	▨	▨	↑ TMAO	■	
Displaces Healthier Foods	■		Uremic Toxins	■	
Less Satiating	■		Dietary Acid Load	■	
↑ Weight Gain	■		Kidney Function	■	

Figure 11

as sodium and TMAO, but LDL cholesterol is "unequivocally recognized as the principal driving force in the development of ASCVD," atherosclerotic cardiovascular disease, our leading cause of death.[834]

Current guidelines suggest we may want to try to get our LDL as low as possible.[835] The title of a review in the *American Journal of Preventive Cardiology* on the importance of lowering LDL put it succinctly: "Lower for Longer Is Better."[836] Even if our LDL is "normal" and even if other heart disease risk factors are considered "optimal,"[837] it is of utmost importance to control it.[838]

If LDL is the primary driver of our primary killer, then if we could know just one thing about any food—if we could ask just one question—it would be: *What does the food do to my LDL cholesterol?*[839] To know that, we can look at nutrition labels for saturated fat, trans fat, and cholesterol, since "any intake level above 0%" of any of the three can increase LDL cholesterol and, therefore, increase risk of our leading cause of death.[840]

Conventional meats are not only a leading source of saturated fat and cholesterol in our diet.[841] With the removal of partially hydrogenated oils from the U.S. food supply,[842] animal products are now the leading dietary source of trans fat as well, as meat and dairy can contain them naturally.[843] Plant-based meat can contain trans fat because some is created in the refining of vegetable oils, but conventional burgers were found to contain twice as many trans fats as plant-based ones.[844]

Online, some bloggers parrot the egg industry's talking point that the 2015 U.S. Dietary Guidelines removed its dietary cholesterol limit,[845] but anyone who actually bothered to read the guidelines would see the cholesterol caution was actually *strengthened*, advising Americans to "eat as little dietary cholesterol as possible" as recommended by the Institute of Medicine, the most prestigious medical body in the United States.[846]

This advice was reiterated in the more recent dietary guidelines: "The National Academies [of Science] recommends that dietary cholesterol consumption be as low as possible."[847] While eggs are, gram for gram, the most concentrated source of cholesterol, the greatest contributor in our diet is meat, including poultry and fish.[848] Since cholesterol is only present in animal-derived foods, it's not surprising that plant-based meats contain no cholesterol (unless they contain cheese or eggs).[849]

The saturated fat content is usually comparatively low in plant-based meats, averaging between half and a third that of their meat matches.[850] In the United States, plant-based burger meat averages seven times lower in saturated fat[851] compared to the most commonly purchased ground beef.[852] For some categories like meatballs, bacon, and deli slices, the *most* saturated-fattiest plant-based meat has less saturated fat than even the *leanest* meat comparator.[853]

When put to the test in randomized controlled trials, replacing conventional meat with plant-based meat significantly lowers intake of saturated fat.[854] Does this translate into a drop in LDL cholesterol? Yes. For example, in the Stanford SWAP-MEAT trial, study participants replaced two and a half servings a day of burgers and beef from cows, sausage from pigs, and breasts from chickens with Beyond Meat's burgers, sausages, and chicken from plants, then vice versa, for eight weeks each, using all organic meats, including grass-fed beef. During the plant-based meat phase, overall saturated fat was significantly lower, so, unsurprisingly, their LDL cholesterol significantly dropped.[855]

The RE-MAP trial also lasted eight weeks but found no LDL benefit. However, instead of replacing two and a half servings a day, participants replaced only about half a single daily serving in the first month and a third of a daily serving in the second month.[856] But, swapping as little as a single serving a day is enough to significantly lower LDL cholesterol.[857]

If we replace all animal protein with an ultra-processed plant-based meat as healthy as TVP, research has shown we can achieve as much as a 50-point drop in our LDL cholesterol within just three weeks.[858] In the same time frame, swapping two daily servings of meat for mycoprotein Quorn products can lower LDL by as much as 38 points compared to control.[859] Even just two weeks of the same swap can significantly reduce LDL.[860] Overall, a meta-analysis of a dozen trials found that replacing at least some meat with plant- or mycoprotein-based meat on a daily basis leads, on average, to a "highly significant" 15-point reduction in LDL cholesterol within an average of six weeks.[861]

Maintaining a 15-point drop in LDL for five years would be expected to reduce risk of heart disease by about 10%. After a dozen years, we'd expect a reduction of more like 15%, and, across 50 years or so, by 25%.[862] Note that this reduction in risk is independent of baseline LDL, meaning we get the same relative reduction in risk even if our LDL is so-called normal, under 100.[863]

The benefit only accrues if our cholesterol stays down, and it turns out that it may even get better. In that unprecedented four-year randomized control trial of a plant-based meat swap, when diabetics were randomized to replace half their animal protein intake with TVP, their LDL continued to go down year after year, ending up 26 points lower than those in the control group.[864] That reduction in LDL cholesterol could net a nearly 40% drop in risk over a lifetime of our number one killer—just by replacing half our animal protein with ultra-processed plant protein.[865]

An estimated 20 million Americans with coronary heart disease are having 800,000 heart attacks a year.[866] If we all started replacing some of our meat with plant-based meat, imagine how many lives could be saved.

The Role of Plant Protein in Reducing Cholesterol

The largest comparative analysis of saturated fat levels, examining more than a thousand products across five countries, concluded that "meat substitutes have great potential in terms of the overall goal of reducing saturated fat intake in the diets, which in turn could reduce the associated detrimental health effects."[867] Instead of swapping a hamburger for a veggie burger, why not just switch to chicken or fish? Because it doesn't work.

A meta-analysis of randomized controlled trials comparing the effects of beef versus poultry and/or fish consumption found no significant difference in terms of LDL cholesterol.[868] An updated meta-analysis of four times as many studies also found there was no benefit from switching from red meat to chicken or other poultry products and that beef was actually better than fish. On average, switching from beef to fish *raised* LDL cholesterol. The researchers attribute this to using particularly lean cuts of beef as the comparator, but even organic grass-fed beef appears to be no match for plant-based meat, as shown in the Stanford SWAP-MEAT trial.[869]

As I've noted, there are some extreme outliers—plant-based meats with *more* saturated fat than conventional meat.[870] So, if a study were designed to replace meat with plant-based meat with similar saturated fat levels, LDL levels might not budge.[871] But the extraordinary study I previously mentioned that netted a 33-point lower LDL compared to control within just three weeks of replacing two daily servings of meat was specifically designed to have no difference in saturated fat.[872] Why did LDL levels improve so much even without a change in saturated fat intake?

Was it the fiber?[873] The daily difference in fiber intake was only about 10 grams,[874] so that would probably account for only an 11-point difference in LDL of the 33-point spread.[875] Something else must be going on. In fact, in the remarkable four-year study that achieved a 26-point LDL drop in those randomized to replace half their animal protein, not only was saturated fat intake not significantly different compared to the control group, but fiber intakes were even lower in the plant-based meat group—yet they still got a potentially life-saving drop in LDL cholesterol.[876]

Was it the dietary cholesterol? Seeing a reduction in LDL despite similar fiber and saturated fat intakes may be partly explained by differences in dietary cholesterol intake.[877] The cholesterol in the meat we eat doesn't raise blood cholesterol levels as much as the meat's saturated fat and trans fats do, but it does still contribute.[878] However, even if saturated animal fat and cholesterol are kept the same—by adding pork, beef, or chicken fat to meat substitutes and essentially giving study participants cholesterol pills to even it all out—researchers sometimes *still* find an advantage in the plant-protein group.[879] Maybe it's the plant protein itself?

We discovered 50 years ago that when straight plant protein is switched to straight animal protein on a low-fat, cholesterol-free diet, the animal protein itself raises cholesterol levels in the blood,[880] but that was in rabbits. Finally, in 2019, the APPROACH trial (Animal and Plant Protein and Cardiovascular Health)—on humans—was published.[881]

Diets based on red meat, white meat, and plant-based meat, as well as less-processed plant proteins like tofu, were matched for saturated fat and fiber.[882] Both red meat and white meat resulted in higher LDL in the otherwise comparable diets, independent of saturated fat and fiber.[883] No cholesterol pills were taken by those in the plant group, so they averaged at least 100 fewer milligrams of cholesterol a day,[884] but that would be expected to decrease blood cholesterol by only about 4 points, and the study showed twice that difference, so there may really be a plant protein effect.[885]

A meta-analysis of more than a hundred randomized controlled trials comparing the effects of replacing animal protein with plant protein found that it decreased LDL cholesterol. Surprisingly, there didn't seem to be a significant difference between whole plant-food sources and protein isolate products, like plant-based meats. This suggests that the cholesterol-lowering effects are attributable at least in part to the plant protein itself, perhaps due to the different amino acid ratios[886] or other cholesterol-lowering plant compounds still present in protein concentrates, like phytosterols.[887] Either way, plant-based meats may improve certain cardiovascular risk factors even when saturated fat and fiber contents are closely matched.[888] However, as I've reviewed, plant-based products also tend to have less saturated fat and more fiber, which, combined, add a bonus benefit.

How Many Lives Might Be Saved
by Plant-Based Meat?

With processed meat officially classified as a known human carcinogen,[889] global nutrition and health organizations flat-out recommend "avoiding processed meat."[890] This includes the World Health Organization,[891] the American Institute for Cancer Research,[892] Harvard School of Public Health,[893] the World Cancer Research Fund,[894] and leading cancer centers, such as Memorial Sloan Kettering[895] and MD Anderson.[896]

However, considering six health outcomes—colorectal cancer, breast cancer, heart disease, type 2 diabetes, and two kinds of stroke—the optimal amount of *unprocessed* red meat may be zero as well.[897] Even just a 30% reduction in both red and processed meats could lead to a million fewer cases of type 2 diabetes, hundreds of thousands of fewer cases of cardiovascular disease, and tens of thousands of fewer cases of cancer and premature death over a decade.[898]

Diets high in red and processed meats are also the two leading causes of diet-related disability in the United States, responsible for more than a million years lived in disability annually—three times more than diets high in sugar-sweetened beverages—and more than two million years of lost life.[899]

How is "high" defined? A diet "high" in processed meat is defined as *any* intake of processed meat.[900] And a diet "high" in red meat? It is also defined as any intake above an average of zero grams per day.[901] Millions of years of life are lost every year in the United States because people are eating more than zero red meat and processed meat.

Higher intake of meat in general, whether red meat, white meat, processed, or unprocessed, is also associated with an increased risk of death from all-causes together.[902] If people replaced about 75% of the meat in their diet with plant-based meat, up to 50,000 lives a year could be saved in higher-income countries.[903]

Though the cost in human life is most important, a switch to plant-based meat could also cut healthcare spending, potentially thousands of dollars per person. In New Zealand, for instance, it was calculated that replacing red and processed meats with ultra-processed plant-based meats would save its healthcare system the equivalent of $13.5 billion USD, though greater benefits would be expected to accrue if people replaced meat with even healthier alternatives like beans. A bean swap would potentially save as much as the equivalent of $18 billion USD, due in part to lower sodium intake.[904]

As I mentioned previously, plant-based meats appear to have comparably high sodium levels as red meat and poultry,[905] though some products are improving. When I was asked by UBS, the largest investment bank in the world, to contribute to its Future of Food report in 2019, I noted that a Beyond Meat burger had 390 milligrams of sodium,[906] which is within the typical 290- to 400-milligram range of conventional burgers in the United States.[907] The 2024 version of the Beyond Burger is 20% lower at 310 milligrams, due to the use of potassium salt, which uses potassium chloride instead of sodium chloride,[908] and Impossible now has a "lite" beef with only 260 milligrams of sodium.[909] Ideally, though, it would be under 180 milligrams, meeting the World Health Organization's recommendation for less than a 1:1 ratio of sodium to calories. In a perfect world, all the foods we eat would have less sodium (in mg) than calories (in kcal), which would approximate the 2,300-milligram upper daily limit recommended by the U.S. Dietary Guidelines.[910]

ULTRA-PROCESSED FOODS

KEEP THE BABY AND THROW OUT THE BATHWATER

The bottom line is that veggie burgers are not Twinkies, even though both are classified as ultra-processed foods. Now there are two directions we can take with that. We can decry the very concept of ultra-processed,[911] or we can take what I would argue is a better tack: Keep the baby and throw out the bathwater. In other words, instead of denying that ultra-processed foods tend to be worse than less-processed foods or that plant-based meats are ultra-processed, we can understand that, despite this classification, plant-based meats are the rare exception in that they not only compare favorably against the foods they were designed to replace,[912] but they could potentially save hundreds of thousands of lives.

There is, however, some merit to the argument that the term *ultra-processed* is not as useful as many have come to think.

Which Ultra-Processed Foods Are Really to Blame?

We know that increased consumption of ultra-processed foods in general has been associated with an increased risk of death and disease. Just a 10% greater intake may increase the risk of diabetes, cardiovascular diseases, obesity, and cancer,[913] and each additional daily serving may increase the risk of dying prematurely by 2%.[914] But does that apply to all categories of ultra-processed foods? The ultra-processed foods category is so expansive that large studies were needed to break it down.

The Framingham Offspring Study confirmed that higher consumption of ultra-processed foods overall is associated with increased risk of cardiovascular disease, but is it because of burgers or bran flakes? In the study, the link between ultra-processed foods and disease was largely driven by sausage, bologna, salami, hot dogs, burgers, and other ultra-processed meats. Breakfast cereals, which are nearly all ultra-processed, was associated with lower risk, presumably because those choosing cereal for breakfast were eating less bacon and eggs.[915]

In another study, this one 30 times larger,[916] the cardiovascular culprits were soft drinks, both regular and diet; meat, specifically burgers, fried chicken, fried fish, and meat pizza; salty snacks like tortilla chips and potato chips; and candy.[917] In the three big Harvard cohorts that followed 200,000 people for decades—the Nurses' Health Study, Nurses' Health Study II, and Health Professionals Follow-Up Study—cardiovascular risk from ultra-processed products was limited to sugar-sweetened beverages and processed red meat, poultry, and fish (like fish sticks). When the researchers excluded soda and meat, the relationship between ultra-processed foods and cardiovascular disease disappeared.[918]

This may be in part because the relationship between ultra-processed foods and high blood pressure appears to be driven largely by soda and meat intake.[919] "Nutritional advice for cardiovascular health should consider differential consequences of group-specific UPF," concluded the Harvard researchers. "Specifically, our findings suggest soft drinks and processed meats should be discouraged."[920]

Vodka is also considered ultra-processed.[921] When researchers tried excluding alcoholic beverages from their analysis, the link between ultra-processed products and a number of cancers became insignificant, suggesting that the alcohol probably drove those associations.[922] However, for colorectal cancer risk, soda, ready-to-heat mixed meals like frozen pizza, and ready-to-eat meat, including poultry and fish, may also play a role.[923] For pancreatic cancer, its association with ultra-processed foods was more an association with meat and meat products and ultra-processed grain products, like donuts, cake, and cookies.[924]

For diabetes, the increase in risk again appears to be driven mostly by animal-based products, along with the ready-to-heat frozen pizza category.[925] What about death?

Harvard researchers discovered that the ultra-processed foods category showing the strongest associations with mortality was ready-to-eat red meat, poultry, and seafood products. The apparent worst ultra-processed foods when it comes to dying specifically from cancer? The meat/poultry/seafood category. The worst when it comes to dying from cardiovascular disease? Meat/poultry/seafood. The worst when it comes to dying from lung diseases, like emphysema? Meat/poultry/seafood. The worst when it comes to dying from neurodegenerative diseases? Ice cream. (There is one ray of sunshine in this study, though. An ultra-processed dessert was associated with *lower* mortality: dark chocolate.) And the worst when it comes to dying from other causes? Meat/poultry/seafood.[926]

So, unsurprisingly, the worst ultra-processed foods when it comes to dying prematurely in general are meat/poultry/seafood. Sweetened beverages appear to be the second worst. So, the researchers concluded that the "major factors contributing to the harmful influence of ultra-processed foods on mortality" may be "meat/poultry/seafood based ready-to-eat products and sugar sweetened and artificially sweetened beverages."[927]

That's what a systematic review and meta-analysis of all such studies showed on ultra-processed foods and all-cause mortality.[928] Put all the studies together, and the only categories of ultra-processed products associated with dying earlier were sweetened beverages and meat. So, when we talk about the negative, life-shortening effects of ultra-processed *food*, we're really only talking about the negative, life-shortening effects of ultra-processed meat, like burgers, chicken nuggets, and fish sticks.[929]

Plant-Based Meats and Milks Linked to Less Disease

Though meat appears to be the primary reason ultra-processed foods shorten people's lives,[930] the association between greater ultra-processed foods intake and higher mortality appears to be present even among vegetarians.[931] Yes, plant-based diets have been linked to a reduced risk of a variety of deadly diseases, but that doesn't mean we can live off vegan donuts. A study of more than 100,000 Brits found that while *non*-ultra-processed plant foods, like fruits and vegetables, are associated with lower risk of disease, ultra-processed "plant-origin" products like Oreos and Mountain Dew are, not surprisingly, associated with higher risks.[932] What was surprising, however, was how these study findings were reported in the mainstream media.

The Telegraph ran the headline: "The Hidden Health Hazards of Vegan Sausages."[933] *The Daily Mail* went with "Vegan Fake Meats Are Linked to Increase in Heart Deaths...."[934] What? I thought the study was about junk food. Indeed, if the reporters had bothered to look at the study, they would have seen that plant-based meats made up only 0.2% of the participants' diet. About 40% of their diet was composed of ultra-processed plant-origin foods, but only about 1/500th of their intake was plant-based meat. Those in the study were eating 30 times more pastries. Aren't those more likely to be the culprit? They ate 14 times more french fries and candy and drank four times more hard liquor.[935] But how much click bait can the media get if it just tells people to lay off the whisky and cream puffs?

The only way conclusions about specific products like plant-based meat can be drawn is to run a more granular analysis and separate them out. One study out of France on obesity had an eclectic category of "ultra-processed fruits and vegetables" that included meat alternatives along with powdered soup and fruit compote for which no link was found. Obesity was tied only to ultra-processed animal products, fats, and beverages.[936] However, to fully separate out plant-based meats, we'd need a study of epic proportions. Enter: the EPIC study.

The European Prospective Investigation into Cancer and Nutrition (EPIC) study followed more than a quarter-million people for more than a decade.[937] As usual, higher consumption of ultra-processed foods in general was associated with increased risk of diseases like heart disease and cancer, but the study was able to drill down to find the true culprits. The only categories of ultra-processed foods linked to disease were, once again, animal products and sweetened beverages. Specifically *not* associated with risk was plant-based meat.[938]

The researchers concluded "our results suggest that higher consumption of UPF increases the risk of cancer and cardiometabolic multimorbidity."[939] But, as commentators pointed out, "their data only show that consumption of foods of animal origin and sugary or artificially sweetened beverages is associated with such a risk."[940] When the original researchers were challenged to go back and exclude the animal-based foods and beverages, the relationship between ultra-processed foods and those diseases disappeared.[941]

Notably, when it came to ultra-processed foods and diabetes, plant-based meats and milks appeared to cut the risk of developing diabetes in half. Based on hundreds of thousands of people followed for more than a decade, animal products were associated with more than twice the risk. In contrast, plant-based alternatives appeared protective, linked to less than half the risk of developing diabetes.[942]

The only other population study of ultra-processed foods that separated out plant-based meats looked at telomere length, which is used to measure cellular aging. Researchers found that a higher consumption of ultra-processed foods in general was associated with a shorter telomere length, a sign of accelerated aging; however, some categories, like breakfast cereals, were associated with *longer* telomere length, suggesting *slower* aging. And the class of foods associated with the longest telomeres? Plant-based meat.[943]

There have been previous observational studies on plant-based meat. The Adventist Health Study-2 found that those who ate plant-based meat daily appeared to cut their risk of hip fracture in half, compared to those eating it less than once a week.[944] In the original Adventist study, schoolchildren who ate plant-based meats appeared to have half the odds of being overweight, compared to those eating animal-based meat. (*Whole* sources of plant protein did even better, associated with only a quarter the odds.)[945] Girls who eat more meat start their periods at an earlier age, which may help explain why childhood meat consumption is linked to breast cancer later in life, since the earlier you start your period, the higher your lifetime risk.[946] In contrast, girls eating plant-based meat are able to, on average, delay the onset of menstruation by nine months.[947]

Observational studies like these cannot prove cause and effect, but randomized, controlled, interventional trials lasting up to four years documented throughout this book demonstrate that, compared to conventional meat, plant-based meat can offer a range of nutritional benefits, lower LDL cholesterol and triglycerides, bolster satiety, facilitate weight loss, enhance blood sugar control, improve newborn outcomes in gestational diabetes, reduce acid reflux and heartburn symptoms, better support the gut microbiome, decrease inflammation, strengthen artery function, reduce oxidative stress, trim TMAO and other uremic toxins, and improve overall kidney function.

Saving 100,000 Lives with Soy Milk

What about ultra-processed plant-based eggs and dairy? "Besides plant-based meat substitutes," wrote the director of the Stroke Prevention & Atherosclerosis Research Centre, "there is great potential for reduction of cardiovascular risk with the use of egg substitutes." This makes sense, given the evidence that eggs can increase the levels of TMAO[948] and cholesterol in our blood,[949] but there have yet to be any randomized controlled trials swapping eggs from hens for eggs from plants. However, there have been a surprising number of interventional trials on substituting soy milk for dairy milk.[950]

Consumers evidently prefer oat and almond milks, but soy milk is the healthiest.[951] It's the only plant-based milk that passes a series of nutrient standards.[952] One thing it isn't fortified with, though, is iodine.[953] Dairy milk contains the essential mineral because iodine supplements are fed to cows and iodine-containing antibacterials are applied to their teats, and the disinfectants apparently leach into their milk.[954] Why doesn't the plant-based milk industry add iodine, too? Good question. The reluctance is attributed to the "[l]ack of awareness about the importance of iodine in the diet...."[955]

Plant-based milks with added sugar may also be at a dental disadvantage,[956] though some studies show that plant-based milks are preferable to dairy milk. Researchers compared seven different types of plant-based milks and measured how much biofilm built up in vitro by the dental plaque–forming bacteria that cause cavities. The worst was a chocolate cashew milk, but cow's milk, used as a control, yielded more than five times more biofilm than all of them.[957] Another study, however, showed sweetened soy milk to be just as biofilm-forming.[958] Sweetened soy milk may be more acidogenic, better at feeding the cavity-forming bacteria.[959] This can then translate into greater demineralization of tooth enamel. So soy milk with added sugar is likely to be a cavity risk.[960] Dairy milk naturally contains sugar, but the milk sugar lactose has been shown to be less cavity-producing than the sucrose table sugar that is added to foods.[961] So, for the milk that best lowers cholesterol without contributing to excess cavity risk, we should choose unsweetened soy milk.[962]

Based on 17 randomized controlled trials, drinking soy milk instead of cow's milk results in significant improvements in blood pressure, cholesterol, and inflammation—an 8-point drop in systolic blood pressure, a 5-point drop in diastolic blood pressure, a 7-point drop in LDL cholesterol, and a reduction in the systemic inflammation marker C-reactive protein.[963] Over a lifetime, that 7-point drop in LDL could drop our risk of heart disease by more than 10%—just from switching milks.[964] If all the dairy in high-income countries were replaced with soy milk, we could potentially reduce overall mortality rates by 4%.[965] That would mean saving the lives of more than 100,000 Americans every year.

PLANT-BASED MEATS VS. WHOLE PLANT FOODS

A review in the American Society for Nutrition journal *Advances in Nutrition* concluded that plant-based meats "are more healthful than the meat they replace but perhaps less so than less-processed forms of plant protein, such as legumes and whole grains." Wait, just *perhaps* less so? Figure 12 shows how plant-based meat compares to whole plant foods.

Yes, plant-based meat is superior in almost every way to conventional meat, but *whole plant foods* not only make up for all the shortfalls—they do even better in many categories. For example, bean-derived plant-based meats may average five times less saturated fat than their meat comparators, but actual beans have *40* times less. Plant-based meat may be no worse on sodium, but legumes, like beans, split peas, chickpeas, and lentils, may be 500 times better.[966] A bean-based burger may have half the trans fat of a meat-based burger, but actual beans have none at all. The five grams of fiber in a bean-based meat are better than the zero grams in regular meat, but the nine grams of fiber in the same serving size of beans are better still.

There are interventional trials that demonstrate the greater benefits of whole plant foods. For example, there was typically no difference in blood sugar control or inflammation when comparing meat with most plant-based meats, but when people replaced two daily servings of meat, three days a week, with lentils, chickpeas, peas, or beans, they got a

Conventional Meat vs. Ultra-Processed Plant-Based Meat vs. Whole Plants

Legend:

★	Even better
(white)	Usually better
(gray)	About the same
(black)	Usually worse

	MEAT	PLANT-BASED MEAT	WHOLE PLANTS		MEAT	PLANT-BASED MEAT	WHOLE PLANTS
Nutrient Profile	■		★	↑ IR (vs. TVP)	■		★
Saturated Fat	■		★	↑ IR (vs. Others)	▨	▨	
Trans Fat	■		★	Heartburn	■		★
Cholesterol	■			↑ Gut Dysbiosis	■		★
Fiber	■		★	↑ Inflammation (vs. TVP)	■		★
Calorie Density	■		★	↑ Inflammation (vs. Other)	▨	▨	
Softer Texture	▨	▨		↑ Endothelial Dysfunction	■		★
De-Encapsulated Calories				↑ Oxidative Stress	■		★
Phytonutrients	■		★	Salmonella	■		
Antioxidants	■		★	Campylobacter	■		
AGEs (ELISA)	■		★	Toxoplasma	■		
AGEs (UPLC)	▨	▨		Antibiotic Resistance	■		
Furosine	▨	▨		Antibiotic Residues	■		
Acrylamide	▨	▨		Hormones	■		
HCAs	■			Pollutants	■		
PAHs	■			Mold Toxins		■	
Nitrates	■			Food Allergens		■	
Salt	▨	▨		Carcinogen Status	■		
Sugar	▨	▨		Neu5gc	■		
Emulsifiers		■	★	↑ IGF-1	▨	▨	
Packaging Chemicals	▨	▨		↑ TMAO	■		
Displaces Healthier Foods	■		★	Uremic Toxins	■		
Less Satiating	■		★	Dietary Acid Load	■		★
↑ Weight Gain	■		★	Kidney Function	■		★

Figure 12

significant improvement in all three inflammatory markers that were measured, C-reactive protein, interleukin 6, and tumor necrosis factor,[967] as well as lower fasting blood sugars and improved insulin sensitivity.[968]

Ultra-processed plant protein can beat out conventional meat, but whole soybeans can beat out both. A randomized crossover trial replaced one serving of meat a day with either TVP or soy nuts, which are roasted whole soybeans. The ultra-processed soy improved insulin resistance, but the whole soy food improved it even more, such that there was a significant decrease in fasting blood sugars in the soy nut group, but not the soy protein group. The soy meat significantly lowered LDL, but the *soybeans* lowered it even more.[969]

Meat Methadone

In a sense, the comparisons to legumes are irrelevant if people aren't going to eat them.[970] Yes, nutrition policies and dietary guidelines should continue to emphasize a diet rich in whole plant-based foods,[971] but we shouldn't let the perfect be the enemy of the good. Plant-based meat alternatives are better than the alternative.

Indeed, if all meat in high-income countries were replaced with whole legumes, we could potentially decrease mortality rates by 5% or 6%.[972] That could mean saving 180,000 lives every year in the United States. If we instead replaced conventional meat with processed or ultra-processed plant-based meat, we'd save only about 130,000 American lives a year, about a 4% drop in overall mortality.

That's still more than 100,000 lives saved every year.

With their added saturated fat and sodium, plant-based meats are not exactly healthy, but they are *healthier*. They are healthier than the foods they were designed to replace. They are better, but not the best. That's why you'll hear leading voices, like the past chair of nutrition at Harvard, saying, yes, they may be better than meat, but the best option would be whole foods.[973] Michael Pollen was acknowledged in the original ultra-processed paper by Professor Monteiro.[974] Famous for his quote, "Eat food. Not too much. Mostly plants," Pollen was asked about the Impossible Burger and replied that he thought it was an excellent product. Not real food, he said, but that doesn't mean he's against it.[975]

Even Professor Monteiro acknowledged that plant-based meat can be a case in which the ultra-processed foods are better than their less-processed alternatives, though he was similarly concerned that plant-based burgers might displace even healthier whole plant foods.[976] That might be true for those rare individuals already eating a healthy plant-based diet, but about 9 out of 10 people buying these products would be otherwise eating meat, so, for them, it's a much healthier choice.[977] Plant-based meat might be considered "meat *with benefits*."[978]

Plant-based meats are not designed to replace whole plant foods but, instead, offer a stepping stone in the transition away from conventional meat.[979] The hope is that plant-based meats will lead to the greater consumption of whole plant foods. As Christopher Gardner, the head of Stanford Nutrition Studies Research Group, put it: "I'm hoping that plant-based meats will be a gateway drug to legumes."[980]

CONCLUSION

The most important question in nutrition may be *compared to what?*[981] A scientific consensus of leading nutrition experts strongly endorsed the "compared to what" approach: "What we consume *and* what we don't consume instead, both contribute to health outcomes."[982]

Eating is kind of a zero-sum game. Every food has an opportunity cost. Every time we put something in our mouth, it's a lost opportunity to put something even healthier in our mouth. So, if we want to know if something is healthy, we have to compare it to what we would have eaten instead.

For example, are eggs healthy? Compared to what? Compared to breakfast sausage, yes. Sausage and other processed meats are known human carcinogens. Each 50-gram serving a day, which is like a single breakfast sausage link, is linked to an 18% higher risk of colorectal cancer,[983] the number one cancer killer of nonsmokers. So, the risk of getting colorectal cancer from eating one sausage link a day is about the same as the increased risk of lung cancer we'd get from breathing secondhand smoke all day living with a smoking spouse.[984] Compared to sausage, eggs are a better choice, but compared to oatmeal, eggs are not.

Are ultra-processed plant-based meats healthy?[985] Compared to the meat products they were designed to replace? The answer is clearly *yes*. In fact, if you remember, a systematic review and meta-analysis of all the best studies on ultra-processed foods and mortality, involving more than five million people, found that only two ultra-processed products were linked to a shortened lifespan: sweetened beverages and meat. So, the only ultra-processed *food* that appears to be killing people is meat.[986] In that case, instead of being a contributor, plant-based meats may be the *solution* to the ultra-processed foods problem.

ACKNOWLEDGMENTS

Thanks to Paul Shapiro and Bruce Friedrich for their critical feedback on my manuscript and for writing the two seminal books in the field. Paul published *Clean Meat* in 2018, and Bruce's *Meat* will be out in early 2026.

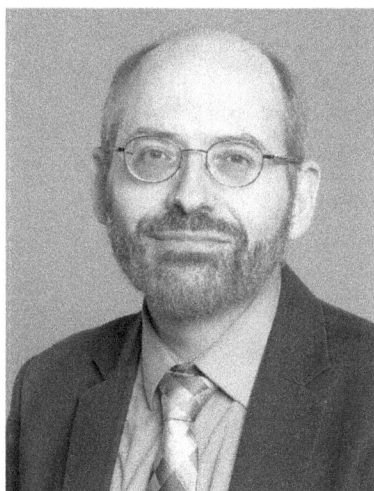

A founding member and fellow of the American College of Life-style Medicine, MICHAEL GREGER, M.D., FACLM is a physician, *New York Times* bestselling author, internationally recognized speaker on nutrition, and founder of the acclaimed nonprofit public health organization NutritionFacts.org. He is a graduate of the Cornell University College of Agriculture and Life Sciences and Tufts University School of Medicine. All proceeds he receives from his books and speaking engagements are donated directly to charity.

NOTES

1   Lawrence M. Ultra-processed foods: a fit-for-purpose concept for nutrition policy activities to tackle unhealthy and unsustainable diets. *Br J Nutr*. 2023;129(12):2195–8. doi: 10.1017/S000711452200280X

2   Sugar as food. *JAMA*. 1913;61(7):492–3. doi: 10.1001/jama.1913.04350070046019

3   Lawrence M. Ultra-processed foods: a fit-for-purpose concept for nutrition policy activities to tackle unhealthy and unsustainable diets. *Br J Nutr*. 2023;129(12):2195–8. doi: 10.1017/S000711452200280X

4   Mozaffarian D, Rosenberg I, Uauy R. History of modern nutrition science—implications for current research, dietary guidelines, and food policy. *BMJ*. 2018;361:k2392. doi: 10.1136/bmj.k2392

5   Jacobs DR, Tapsell LC. Food, not nutrients, is the fundamental unit in nutrition. *Nutr Rev*. 2008;65(10):439–50. doi: 10.1111/j.1753-4887.2007.tb00269.x

6   Lawrence M. Ultra-processed foods: a fit-for-purpose concept for nutrition policy activities to tackle unhealthy and unsustainable diets. *Br J Nutr*. 2023;129(12):2195–8. doi: 10.1017/S000711452200280X

7   Ridgway E, Baker P, Woods J, Lawrence M. Historical developments and paradigm shifts in public health nutrition science, guidance and policy actions: a narrative review. *Nutrients*. 2019;11(3):531. doi:10.3390/nu11030531

8   Vadiveloo MK, Gardner CD. Not all ultra-processed foods are created equal: a case for advancing research and policy that balances health and nutrition security. *Diabetes Care*. 2023;46(7):1327–9. doi: 10.2337/dci23-0018

9   Anastasiou K, Ribeiro De Melo P, Slater S, et al. From harmful nutrients to ultra-processed foods: exploring shifts in 'foods to limit' terminology used in national food-based dietary guidelines. *Public Health Nutr*. 2023;26(11):2539–50. doi: 10.1017/S1368980022002580

10 Monteiro CA. Nutrition and health. The issue is not food, nor nutrients, so much as processing. *Public Health Nutr*. 2009;12(5):729–31. doi: 10.1017/S1368980009005291

11   Touvier M, da Costa Louzada ML, Mozaffarian D, Baker P, Juul F, Srour B. Ultra-processed foods and cardiometabolic health: public health policies to reduce consumption cannot wait. *BMJ*. 2023;383:e075294. doi: 10.1136/bmj-2023-075294

12   Organic Quinoa, Kale & Red Lentil soup. Amy's Kitchen. Accessed April 21, 2025. https://www.amys.com/our-foods/organic-quinoa-kale-red-lentil-soup

13   Lipton Recipe Soup & Dip Mix, Vegetable. Publix. Accessed September 29, 2025. https://delivery.publix.com/landing?product_id=76912&retailer_id=57&postal_code=30248&region_id=7767136496

14   Indomie instant noodles soup vegetable flavour. Indomie. Accessed April 21, 2025. https://www.indomie.hr/en/products/indomie-instant-noodles-soup-vegetable-flavour/

15   Shredded Wheat® Original. Nestlé. Accessed April 21, 2025. https://www.nestle-cereals.com/uk/brands/shredded-wheat/original

16   Marshmallow Fruity Pebbles™ cereal. Post Consumer Brands. Accessed April 21, 2025. https://www.postconsumerbrands.com/brands/pebbles/products/marshmallow-fruity-pebbles-cereal/

17   Monteiro CA, Cannon G, Moubarac JC, Levy RB, Louzada MLC, Jaime PC. The UN Decade of Nutrition, the NOVA food classification and the trouble with ultra-processing. *Public Health Nutr*. 2018;21(1):5–17. doi: 10.1017/S1368980017000234

18   Crimarco A, Landry MJ, Gardner CD. Ultra-processed foods, weight gain, and co-morbidity risk. *Curr Obes Rep*. 2021;11(3):80–92. doi: 10.1007/s13679-021-00460-y

19   Martínez Steele E, Baraldi LG, Louzada ML da C, Moubarac JC, Mozaffarian D, Monteiro CA. Ultra-processed foods and added sugars in the US diet: evidence from a nationally representative cross-sectional study. *BMJ Open*. 2016;6(3):e009892. doi: 10.1136/bmjopen-2015-009892

20   Frosted Wildlicious Wild Berry Pop-Tarts®. Kellanova. Accessed September 29, 2025. https://www.kellanovaus.com/us/en/brands/pop-tarts/pop-tarts-frosted-wildlicious-wild-berry.html

21   Harrison R, Warburton V, Lux A, Atan D. Blindness caused by a junk food diet. *Ann Intern Med*. 2019;171(11):859–61. doi: 10.7326/L19-0361

22   Cotter T, Kotov A, Wang S, Murukutla N. 'Warning: ultra-processed'—a call for warnings on foods that aren't really foods. *BMJ Glob Health*. 2021;6(12):e007240. doi: 10.1136/bmjgh-2021-007240

23   Monteiro CA, Cannon G, Moubarac JC, Levy RB, Louzada MLC, Jaime PC. The UN Decade of Nutrition, the NOVA food classification and the trouble with ultra-processing. *Public Health Nutr*. 2018;21(1):5–17. doi: 10.1017/S1368980017000234

24   O'Connor LE, Higgins KA, Smiljanec K, et al. Perspective: a research roadmap about ultra-processed foods and human health for the United States food system: proceedings from an interdisciplinary, multi-stakeholder workshop. *Adv Nutr*. 2023;14(6):1255–69. doi: 10.1016/j.advnut.2023.09.005

25   Monteiro CA. Nutrition and health. The issue is not food, nor nutrients, so much as processing. *Public Health Nutr*. 2009;12(5):729–31. doi: 10.1017/S1368980009005291

26   Assaf S, Park J, Chowdhry N, et al. Unraveling the evolutionary diet mismatch and its contribution to the deterioration of body composition. *Metabolites*. 2024;14(7):379. doi: 10.3390/metabo14070379

27   Monteiro CA, Cannon G, Moubarac JC, Levy RB, Louzada MLC, Jaime PC. The UN Decade of Nutrition, the NOVA food classification and the trouble with ultra-processing. *Public Health Nutr.* 2018;21(1):5–17. doi:10.1017/S1368980017000234

28   Monteiro CA. Letters to the editor. *Public Health Nutr.* 2009;12(10):1968–9. doi: 10.1017/S1368980009991212

29   Sherling DH, Hennekens CH, Ferris AH. Newest updates to health providers on the hazards of ultra-processed foods and proposed solutions. *Am J Med.* 2024;137(5):395–8. doi: 10.1016/j.amjmed.2024.02.001

30   Touvier M, da Costa Louzada ML, Mozaffarian D, Baker P, Juul F, Srour B. Ultra-processed foods and cardiometabolic health: public health policies to reduce consumption cannot wait. *BMJ.* 2023;383:e075294. doi: 10.1136/bmj-2023-075294

31   Lane MM, Gamage E, Du S, et al. Ultra-processed food exposure and adverse health outcomes: umbrella review of epidemiological meta-analyses. *BMJ.* 2024;384. doi: 10.1136/bmj-2023-077310

32   Cascaes AM, Silva NRJ da, Fernandez M dos S, Bomfim RA, Vaz J dos S. Ultra-processed food consumption and dental caries in children and adolescents: a systematic review and meta-analysis. *Br J Nutr.* 2023;129(8):1370–9. doi: 10.1017/S0007114522002409

33   Wang Z, Lu C, Wang Y, et al. Association between ultra-processed foods consumption and the risk of hypertension: an umbrella review of systematic reviews. *Hellenic J Cardiol.* 2024;76:99–109. doi: 10.1016/j.hjc.2023.07.010

34   Yuan L, Hu H, Li T, et al. Dose–response meta-analysis of ultra-processed food with the risk of cardiovascular events and all-cause mortality: evidence from prospective cohort studies. *Food Funct.* 2023;14(6):2586–96. doi: 10.1039/d2fo02628g

35   Moradi S, Entezari MH, Mohammadi H, et al. Ultra-processed food consumption and adult obesity risk: a systematic review and dose-response meta-analysis. *Crit Rev Food Sci Nutr.* 2023;63(2):249–60. doi: 10.1080/10408398.2021.1946005

36   Dicken SJ, Batterham RL. Ultra-processed food and obesity: what is the evidence? *Curr Nutr Rep.* 2024;13(1):23–38. doi: 10.1007/s13668-024-00517-z

37   Isaksen IM, Dankel SN. Ultra-processed food consumption and cancer risk: a systematic review and meta-analysis. *Clin Nutr.* 2023;42(6):919–28. doi: 10.1016/j.clnu.2023.03.018

38   Henney AE, Gillespie CS, Alam U, Hydes TJ, Mackay CE, Cuthbertson DJ. High intake of ultra-processed food is associated with dementia in adults: a systematic review and meta-analysis of observational studies. *J Neurol.* 2024;271(1):198–210. doi: 10.1007/s00415-023-12033-1

39   Babaei A, Pourmotabbed A, Talebi S, et al. The association of ultra-processed food consumption with adult inflammatory bowel disease risk: a systematic review and dose-response meta-analysis of 4 035 694 participants. *Nutr Rev.* 2024;82(7):861–71. doi: 10.1093/nutrit/nuad101

40   Wu S, Yang Z, Liu S, Zhang Q, Zhang S, Zhu S. Ultra-processed food consumption and long-term risk of irritable bowel syndrome: a large-scale prospective cohort study. *Clin Gastroenterol Hepatol.* 2024;22(7):1497–1507.e5. doi: 10.1016/j.cgh.2024.01.040

41   Xiao B, Huang J, Chen L, et al. Ultra-processed food consumption and the risk of incident chronic kidney disease: a systematic review and meta-analysis of cohort studies. *Ren Fail.* 2024;46(1):2306224. doi: 10.1080/0886022X.2024.2306224

42   Lane MM, Gamage E, Du S, et al. Ultra-processed food exposure and adverse health outcomes: umbrella review of epidemiological meta-analyses. *BMJ*. 2024;384. doi: 10.1136/bmj-2023-077310

43   Dai S, Wellens J, Yang N, et al. Ultra-processed foods and human health: an umbrella review and updated meta-analyses of observational evidence. *Clin Nutr*. 2024;43(6):1386–94. doi: 10.1016/j.clnu.2024.04.016

44   Dai S, Wellens J, Yang N, et al. Ultra-processed foods and human health: an umbrella review and updated meta-analyses of observational evidence. *Clin Nutr*. 2024;43(6):1386–94. doi: 10.1016/j.clnu.2024.04.016

45   Lane MM, Gamage E, Travica N, et al. Ultra-processed food consumption and mental health: a systematic review and meta-analysis of observational studies. *Nutrients*. 2022;14(13):2568. doi: 10.3390/nu14132568

46   Lane MM, Gamage E, Travica N, et al. Ultra-processed food consumption and mental health: a systematic review and meta-analysis of observational studies. *Nutrients*. 2022;14(13):2568. doi: 10.3390/nu14132568

47   Fransen HP, Boer JMA, Beulens JWJ, et al. Associations between lifestyle factors and an unhealthy diet. *Eur J Public Health*. 2017;27(2):274–8. doi:10.1093/eurpub/ckw190

48   Kesse E, Clavel-Chapelon F, Slimani N, van Liere M; E3N Group. Do eating habits differ according to alcohol consumption? Results of a study of the French cohort of the European Prospective Investigation into Cancer and Nutrition (E3N-EPIC). *Am J Clin Nutr*. 2001;74(3):322–7. doi:10.1093/ajcn/74.3.322

49   Barbaresko J, Bröder J, Conrad J, Szczerba E, Lang A, Schlesinger S. Ultra-processed food consumption and human health: an umbrella review of systematic reviews with meta-analyses. *Crit Rev Food Sci Nutr*. 2025;65(11):1999–2007. doi: 10.1080/10408398.2024.2317877

50   Visioli F, Marangoni F, Fogliano V, et al. The ultra-processed foods hypothesis: a product processed well beyond the basic ingredients in the package. *Nutr Res Rev*. 2023;36(2):340–50. doi: 10.1017/S0954422422000117

51   Lane MM, Gamage E, Du S, et al. Ultra-processed food exposure and adverse health outcomes: umbrella review of epidemiological meta-analyses. *BMJ*. 2024;384. doi: 10.1136/bmj-2023-077310

52   Bestari FF, Andarwulan N, Palupi E. Synthesis of effect sizes on dose response from ultra-processed food consumption against various noncommunicable diseases. *Foods*. 2023;12(24):4457. doi: 10.3390/foods12244457

53   Dicken SJ, Batterham RL. The role of diet quality in mediating the association between ultra-processed food intake, obesity and health-related outcomes: a review of prospective cohort studies. *Nutrients*. 2021;14(1):23. doi: 10.3390/nu14010023

54   Monteiro CA. Letters to the editor. *Public Health Nutr*. 2009;12(10):1968–9. doi: 10.1017/S136898000999139X

55   Dicken SJ, Batterham RL. The role of diet quality in mediating the association between ultra-processed food intake, obesity and health-related outcomes: a review of prospective cohort studies. *Nutrients*. 2021;14(1):23. doi: 10.3390/nu14010023

56   Dicken SJ, Batterham RL. The role of diet quality in mediating the association between ultra-processed food intake, obesity and health-related outcomes: a review of prospective cohort studies. *Nutrients*. 2021;14(1):23. doi: 10.3390/nu14010023

57   Dunford EK, Popkin B, Ng SW. Junk food intake among adults in the United States. *J Nutr*. 2022;152(2):492–500. doi: 10.1093/jn/nxab205

58   Vlassopoulos A, Katidi A, Noutsos S, Kapsokefalou M. Precision food composition data as a tool to decipher the riddle of ultra-processed foods and nutritional quality. *Foods*. 2024;13(8):1259. doi: 10.3390/foods13081259

59   Scrinis G, Monteiro C. From ultra-processed foods to ultra-processed dietary patterns. *Nat Food*. 2022;3(9):671–3. doi: 10.1038/s43016-022-00599-4

60   Menichetti F, Leone A. Consumption of ultra-processed foods and health harm. *Nutrients*. 2023;15(13):2945. doi: 10.3390/nu15132945

61   Diet Coke. The Coca-Cola Company. Accessed September 27, 2025. https://www.coca-cola.com/us/en/brands/diet-coke/products

62   Smith TJ, Wolfson JA, Jiao D, et al. Caramel color in soft drinks and exposure to 4-methylimidazole: a quantitative risk assessment. *PLoS One*. 2015;10(2):e0118138. doi: 10.1371/journal.pone.0118138

63   IARC Working Group on the Evaluation of Carcinogenic Risks to Humans. *Some Chemicals Present in Industrial and Consumer Products, Food and Drinking-Water*. International Agency for Research on Cancer; 2013. IARC Monographs on the Evaluation of Carcinogenic Risks to Humans, No 101. https://www.ncbi.nlm.nih.gov/books/NBK373192/

64   Diet Coke. The Coca-Cola Company. Accessed September 27, 2025. https://www.coca-cola.com/us/en/brands/diet-coke/products

65   Riboli E, Beland FA, Lachenmeier DW, et al. Carcinogenicity of aspartame, methyleugenol, and isoeugenol. *Lancet Oncology*. 2023;24(8):848–50. doi: 10.1016/S1470-2045(23)00341-8

66   Diet Coke. The Coca-Cola Company. Accessed September 27, 2025. https://www.coca-cola.com/us/en/brands/diet-coke/products

67   Ritz E, Hahn K, Ketteler M, Kuhlmann MK, Mann J. Phosphate additives in food—a health risk. *Dtsch Arztebl Int*. 2012;109(4):49–55. doi: 10.3238/arztebl.2012.0049

68   Calvo MS, Dunford EK, Uribarri J. Industrial use of phosphate food additives: a mechanism linking ultra-processed food intake to cardiorenal disease risk? *Nutrients*. 2023;15(16):3510. doi: 10.3390/nu15163510

69   Diet Coke. The Coca-Cola Company. Accessed September 27, 2025. https://www.coca-cola.com/us/en/brands/diet-coke/products

70   Bateman B, Warner JO, Hutchinson E, et al. The effects of a double blind, placebo controlled, artificial food colourings and benzoate preservative challenge on hyperactivity in a general population sample of preschool children. *Arch Dis Child*. 2004;89(6):506–11. doi: 10.1136/adc.2003.031435

71   Lane MM, Gamage E, Du S, et al. Ultra-processed food exposure and adverse health outcomes: umbrella review of epidemiological meta-analyses. *BMJ*. 2024;384:e077310. doi: 10.1136/bmj-2023-077310

72   Warner JO. Artificial food additives: hazardous to long-term health? *Arch Dis Child*. 2024;109(11):882–5. doi: 10.1136/archdischild-2023-326565

73   Sherling DH, Hennekens CH, Ferris AH. Newest updates to health providers on the hazards of ultra-processed foods and proposed solutions. *Am J Med*. 2024;137(5):395–8. doi: 10.1016/j.amjmed.2024.02.001

74   Trumbo PR, Bleiweiss-Sande R, Campbell JK, et al. Toward a science-based classification of processed foods to support meaningful research and effective health policies. *Front Nutr*. 2024;11:1389601. doi: 10.3389/fnut.2024.1389601

75   *Breast Cancer Prevention Partners v FDA*, 18-71260 (9th Cir 2018).

76   Sanchez-Siles L, Roman S, Fogliano V, Siegrist M. Naturalness and healthiness in "ultra-processed foods": a multidisciplinary perspective and case study. *Trends Food Sci Tech*. 2022;129:667–73. doi: 10.1016/j.tifs.2022.11.009

77   Riboli E, Beland FA, Lachenmeier DW, et al. Carcinogenicity of aspartame, methyleugenol, and isoeugenol. *Lancet Oncology*. 2023;24(8):848–50. doi: 10.1016/S1470-2045(23)00341-8

78   Huff J, LaDou J. Aspartame bioassay findings portend human cancer hazards. *Int J Occup Environ Health*. 2007;13(4):446–8. doi: 10.1179/oeh.2007.13.4.446

79   Soffritti M, Padovani M, Tibaldi E, Falcioni L, Manservisi F, Belpoggi F. The carcinogenic effects of aspartame: the urgent need for regulatory re-evaluation. *Am J Indl Med*. 2014;57(4):383–97. doi: 10.1002/ajim.22296

80   Astrup A, Monteiro CA. Does the concept of "ultra-processed foods" help inform dietary guidelines, beyond conventional classification systems? Debate consensus. *Am J Clin Nutr*. 2022;116(6):1489–91. doi: 10.1093/ajcn/nqac230

81   Greger M. *Seeing Red No. 3: Coloring to Dye For*. NutritionFacts.org. March 10, 2014. Accessed April 14, 2025. https://nutritionfacts.org/video/seeing-red-no-3-coloring-to-dye-for/

82   Termination of provisional listings of color additives. *Fed Regist*. 2023;21 CFR §81.10.

83   Chen A, Kayrala N, Trapeau M, Aoun M, Bordenave N. The clean label trend: an ineffective heuristic that disserves both consumers and the food industry? *Comp Rev Food Sci Food Safe*. 2022;21(6):4921–38. doi: 10.1111/1541-4337.13031

84   Astrup A, Monteiro CA. Does the concept of "ultra-processed foods" help inform dietary guidelines, beyond conventional classification systems? NO. *Am J Clin Nutr*. 2022;116(6):1482–8. doi: 10.1093/ajcn/nqac123

85   Touvier M, da Costa Louzada ML, Mozaffarian D, Baker P, Juul F, Srour B. Ultra-processed foods and cardiometabolic health: public health policies to reduce consumption cannot wait. *BMJ*. 2023;383:e075294. doi:10.1136/bmj-2023-075294

86   Henning RJ, Johnson GT, Coyle JP, Harbison RD. Acrolein can cause cardiovascular disease: a review. *Cardiovasc Toxicol*. 2017;17(3):227–36. doi: 10.1007/s12012-016-9396-5

87   Ewert A, Granvogl M, Schieberle P. Isotope-labeling studies on the formation pathway of acrolein during heat processing of oils. *J Agric Food Chem*. 2014;62(33):8524–9.

88   IARC Working Group on the Identification of Carcinogenic Hazards to Humans. *Acrolein, Crotonaldehyde, and Arecoline*. International Agency for Research on Cancer; 2021. IARC Monographs on the Identification of Carcinogenic Hazards to Humans, No 128. https://www.ncbi.nlm.nih.gov/books/NBK589586/ARC

89   Henning RJ, Johnson GT, Coyle JP, Harbison RD. Acrolein can cause cardiovascular disease: a review. *Cardiovasc Toxicol.* 2017;17(3):227–36. doi: 10.1007/s12012-016-9396-5

90   Nagra M, Tsam F, Ward S, Ur E. Animal vs plant-based meat: a hearty debate. *Can J Cardiol.* 2024;40(7):1198–209. doi: 10.1016/j.cjca.2023.11.005

91   Ewert A, Granvogl M, Schieberle P. Development of two stable isotope dilution assays for the quantitation of acrolein in heat-processed fats. *J Agric Food Chem.* 2011;59(8):3582–9. doi:10.1021/jf200467x

92   Crimarco A, Landry MJ, Gardner CD. Ultra-processed foods, weight gain, and co-morbidity risk. *Curr Obes Rep.* 2021;11(3):80–92. doi: 10.1007/s13679-021-00460-y

93   Eisenreich A, Monien BH, Götz ME, et al. 3-MCPD as contaminant in processed foods: State of knowledge and remaining challenges. *Food Chemistry.* 2023;403:134332. doi: 10.1016/j.foodchem.2022.134332

94   Touvier M, da Costa Louzada ML, Mozaffarian D, Baker P, Juul F, Srour B. Ultra-processed foods and cardiometabolic health: public health policies to reduce consumption cannot wait. *BMJ.* 2023;383:e075294. doi: 10.1136/bmj-2023-075294

95   International Agency for Research on Cancer. *Dry Cleaning, Some Chlorinated Solvents and Other Industrial Chemicals.* Monographs on the Evaluation of Carcinogen Risk to Humans, Vol 63. International Agency for Research on Cancer;1995.

96   International Agency for Research on Cancer. *Some Industrial Chemicals.* Monographs on the Evaluation of Carcinogen Risk to Humans, Vol 60. International Agency for Research on Cancer;1994.

97   Final determination regarding partially hydrogenated oils (removing trans fat). U.S. Food and Drug Administration. October 1, 2024. Accessed October 15, 2025. https://www.fda.gov/food/food-additives-petitions/final-determination-regarding-partially-hydrogenated-oils-removing-trans-fat

98   Touvier M, da Costa Louzada ML, Mozaffarian D, Baker P, Juul F, Srour B. Ultra-processed foods and cardiometabolic health: public health policies to reduce consumption cannot wait. *BMJ.* 2023;383:e075294. doi: 10.1136/bmj-2023-075294

99   Bezelgues JB, Destaillats F. Formation of trans fatty acids during deodorization of edible oils. In: *Trans Fatty Acids in Human Nutrition.* Elsevier; 2012:65–75. doi: 10.1533/9780857097873.65

100   Exler J, Lemar L, Smith L. *Fat and Fatty Acid Content of Selected Foods Containing Trans Fatty Acids, Special Purpose Table No 1.* U.S. Department of Agriculture. 1993. Accessed September 27, 2025. https://www.ars.usda.gov/arsuserfiles/80400525/data/classics/trans_fa.pdf

101   Revealing trans fats. *FDA Consumer.* 2003;37(5):20–6.

102   Liu Y, Yang X, Xiao F, et al. Dietary cholesterol oxidation products: perspectives linking food processing and storage with health implications. *Comp Rev Food Sci Food Safe.* 2022;21(1):738–79. doi: 10.1111/1541-4337.12880

103   Deng C, Li M, Liu Y, et al. Cholesterol oxidation products: potential adverse effect and prevention of their production in foods. *J Agric Food Chem.* 2023;71(48):18645–59. doi: 10.1021/acs.jafc.3c05158

104   Sottero B, Gamba P, Gargiulo S, Leonarduzzi G, Poli G. Cholesterol oxidation products and disease: an emerging topic of interest in medicinal chemistry. *Curr Med Chem*. 2009;16(6):685–705. doi: 10.2174/092986709787458353

105   Maldonado-Pereira L, Schweiss M, Barnaba C, Medina-Meza IG. The role of cholesterol oxidation products in food toxicity. *Food Chem Toxicol*. 2018;118:908–39. doi :10.1016/j.fct.2018.05.059

106   Min JS, Lee SO, Khan MI, et al. Monitoring the formation of cholesterol oxidation products in model systems using response surface methodology. *Lipids Health Dis*. 2015;14(1):77. doi: 10.1186/s12944-015-0074-6

107   Osada K, Hoshina S, Nakamura S, Sugano M. Cholesterol oxidation in meat products and its regulation by supplementation of sodium nitrite and apple polyphenol before processing. *J Agric Food Chem*. 2000;48(9):3823–9. doi: 10.1021/jf991187k

108   Touvier M, da Costa Louzada ML, Mozaffarian D, Baker P, Juul F, Srour B. Ultra-processed foods and cardiometabolic health: public health policies to reduce consumption cannot wait. *BMJ*. 2023;383:e075294. doi: 10.1136/bmj-2023-075294

109   Tian Z, Chen S, Shi Y, Wang P, Wu Y, Li G. Dietary advanced glycation end products (dAGEs): an insight between modern diet and health. *Food Chem*. 2023;415:135735. doi: 10.1016/j.foodchem.2023.135735

110   Green AS. mTOR, glycotoxins and the parallel universe. *Aging (Albany NY)*. 2018;10(12):3654–6. doi: 10.18632/aging.101720

111   Uribarri J, Woodruff S, Goodman S, et al. Advanced glycation end products in foods and a practical guide to their reduction in the diet. *J Am Diet Assoc*. 2010;110(6):911-16.e12. doi: 10.1016/j.jada.2010.03.018

112   Zhang Q, Wang Y, Fu L. Dietary advanced glycation end-products: perspectives linking food processing with health implications. *Comp Rev Food Sci Food Safe*. 2020;19(5):2559–87. doi: 10.1111/1541-4337.12593

113   Uribarri J, Woodruff S, Goodman S, et al. Advanced glycation end products in foods and a practical guide to their reduction in the diet. *J Am Diet Assoc*. 2010;110(6):911-16.e12. doi: 10.1016/j.jada.2010.03.018

114   Uribarri J, Woodruff S, Goodman S, et al. Advanced glycation end products in foods and a practical guide to their reduction in the diet. *J Am Diet Assoc*. 2010;110(6):911-16.e12. doi: 10.1016/j.jada.2010.03.018

115   Touvier M, da Costa Louzada ML, Mozaffarian D, Baker P, Juul F, Srour B. Ultra-processed foods and cardiometabolic health: public health policies to reduce consumption cannot wait. *BMJ*. 2023;383:e075294. doi: 10.1136/bmj-2023-075294

116   Scrinis G, Monteiro C. From ultra-processed foods to ultra-processed dietary patterns. *Nat Food*. 2022;3(9):671–3. doi: 10.1038/s43016-022-00599-4

117   Chen A, Kayrala N, Trapeau M, Aoun M, Bordenave N. The clean label trend: an ineffective heuristic that disserves both consumers and the food industry? *Comp Rev Food Sci Food Safe*. 2022;21(6):4921–38. doi: 10.1111/1541-4337.13031

118   Touvier M, da Costa Louzada ML, Mozaffarian D, Baker P, Juul F, Srour B. Ultra-processed foods and cardiometabolic health: public health policies to reduce consumption cannot wait. *BMJ*. 2023;383:e075294. doi: 10.1136/bmj-2023-075294

119 Tarnow P, Hutzler C, Grabiger S, Schön K, Tralau T, Luch A. Estrogenic activity of mineral oil aromatic hydrocarbons used in printing inks. *PLoS ONE*. 2016;11(1):e0147239. doi: 10.1371/journal.pone.014723

120 Nygaard UC, Vege Å, Rognum T, et al. Toxic effects of mineral oil saturated hydrocarbons (MOSH) and relation to accumulation in rat liver. *Food Chem Toxicol*. 2023;177:113847. doi: 10.1016/j.fct.2023.113847

121 Bevan R, Harrison PTC, Jeffery B, Mitchell D. Evaluating the risk to humans from mineral oils in foods: current state of the evidence. *Food Chem Toxicol*. 2020;136:110966. doi: 10.1016/j.fct.2019.110966

122 Qian S, Ji H, Wu X, et al. Detection and quantification analysis of chemical migrants in plastic food contact products. *PLoS ONE*. 2018;13(12):e0208467. doi: 10.1371/journal. pone.0208467

123 Tumu K, Vorst K, Curtzwiler G. Endocrine modulating chemicals in food packaging: a review of phthalates and bisphenols. *Comp Rev Food Sci Food Safe*. 2023;22(2):1337– 59. doi: 10.1111/1541-4337.13113

124 Rudel RA, Gray JM, Engel CL, et al. Food packaging and bisphenol A and bis(2-ethyhexyl) phthalate exposure: findings from a dietary intervention. *Environ Health Perspect*. 2011;119(7):914–20. doi: 10.1289/ehp.1003170

125 Rowdhwal SSS, Chen J. Toxic effects of di-2-ethylhexyl phthalate: an overview. *Biomed Res Int*. 2018;2018:1750368. doi: 10.1155/2018/1750368

126 Symeonides C, Aromataris E, Mulders Y, et al. An umbrella review of meta-analyses evaluating associations between human health and exposure to major classes of plastic-associated chemicals. *Ann Glob Health*. 2024;90(1):52. doi: 10.5334/aogh.4459.

127 Chen A, Kayrala N, Trapeau M, Aoun M, Bordenave N. The clean label trend: an ineffective heuristic that disserves both consumers and the food industry? *Comp Rev Food Sci Food Safe*. 2022;21(6):4921–38. doi: 10.1111/1541-4337.13031

128 Vom Saal FS, Vandenberg LN. Update on the health effects of bisphenol A: overwhelming evidence of harm. *Endocrinology*. 2021;162(3):bqaa171. doi: 10.1210/endocr/bqaa171

129 Calafat AM, Ye X, Wong LY, Reidy JA, Needham LL. Exposure of the U.S. population to bisphenol A and 4-tertiary-octylphenol: 2003-2004. *Environ Health Perspect*. 2008;116(1):39–44. doi: 10.1289/ehp.10753

130 Carwile JL, Ye X, Zhou X, Calafat AM, Michels KB. Canned soup consumption and urinary bisphenol A: a randomized crossover trial. *JAMA*. 2011;306(20):2218–20. doi: 10.1001/jama.2011.1721.

131 Martínez Steele E, Khandpur N, da Costa Louzada ML, Monteiro CA. Association between dietary contribution of ultra-processed foods and urinary concentrations of phthalates and bisphenol in a nationally representative sample of the US population aged 6 years and older. *PLoS ONE*. 2020;15(7):e0236738. doi: 10.1371/journal. pone.0236738

132 Cao XL, Kosarac I, Popovic S, Zhou S, Smith D, Dabeka R. LC-MS/MS analysis of bisphenol S and five other bisphenols in total diet food samples. *Food Addit Contam Part A Chem Anal Control Expo Risk Assess*. 2019;36(11):1740–7. doi: 10.1080/19440049.2019.1643042

133 Serrano SE, Braun J, Trasande L, Dills R, Sathyanarayana S. Phthalates and diet: a review of the food monitoring and epidemiology data. *Environ Health*. 2014;13(1):43. doi: 10.1186/1476-069X-13-43

134 Ji K, Lim Kho Y, Park Y, Choi K. Influence of a five-day vegetarian diet on urinary levels of antibiotics and phthalate metabolites: a pilot study with "Temple Stay" participants. *Environ Res*. 2010;110(4):375–82. doi: 10.1016/j.envres.2010.02.008

135 Cao XL, Kosarac I, Popovic S, Zhou S, Smith D, Dabeka R. LC-MS/MS analysis of bisphenol S and five other bisphenols in total diet food samples. *Food Addit Contam Part A Chem Anal Control Expo Risk Assess*. 2019;36(11):1740–7. doi: 10.1080/19440049.2019.1643042

136 Steele L, Drummond E, Nishida C, et al. Ending trans fat—the first-ever global elimination program for a noncommunicable disease risk factor. *J Am Coll Cardiol*. 2024;84(7):663–74. doi: 10.1016/j.jacc.2024.04.067

137 Wang Q, Afshin A, Yakoob MY, et al. Impact of nonoptimal intakes of saturated, polyunsaturated, and trans fat on global burdens of coronary heart disease. *JAHA*. 2016;5(1):e002891. doi: 10.1161/JAHA.115.002891

138 Amico A, Wootan MG, Jacobson MF, Leung C, Willett AW. The demise of artificial trans fat: a history of a public health achievement. *Milbank Quarterly*. 2021;99(3):746–70. doi: 10.1111/1468-0009.12515

139 Kelly OJ. Ultraprocessed food is not a replacement for whole food. *Adv Nutr*. 2023;14(5):1244–5. doi: 10.1016/j.advnut.2023.05.016

140 The history of Lucky Charms. General Mills Inc. Accessed September 27, 2025. https://www.generalmills.com/news/stories/the-history-of-lucky-charms

141 Valicente VM, Peng CH, Pacheco KN, et al. Ultraprocessed foods and obesity risk: a critical review of reported mechanisms. *Adv Nutr*. 2023;14(4):718–38. doi: 10.1016/j.advnut.2023.04.006

142 Kelly OJ. Ultraprocessed food is not a replacement for whole food. *Adv Nutr*. 2023;14(5):1244–5. doi: 10.1016/j.advnut.2023.05.016

143 Wiss DA, LaFata EM. Ultra-processed foods and mental health: where do eating disorders fit into the puzzle? *Nutrients*. 2024;16(12):1955. doi: 10.3390/nu16121955

144 Williamson G, Holst B. Dietary reference intake (DRI) value for dietary polyphenols: are we heading in the right direction? *Br J Nutr*. 2008;99(S3):S55–8. doi: 10.1017/S0007114508006867

145 Barabási AL, Menichetti G, Loscalzo J. The unmapped chemical complexity of our diet. *Nat Food*. 2019;1(1):33–7. doi: 10.1038/s43016-019-0005-1

146 Meccariello R, D'Angelo S. Impact of polyphenolic-food on longevity: an elixir of life. An overview. *Antioxidants*. 2021;10(4):507. doi: 10.3390/antiox10040507

147 Assaf S, Park J, Chowdhry N, et al. Unraveling the evolutionary diet mismatch and its contribution to the deterioration of body composition. *Metabolites*. 2024;14(7):379. doi: 10.3390/metabo14070379

148 Leitão AE, Roschel H, Oliveira-Júnior G, et al. Association between ultra-processed food and flavonoid intakes in a nationally representative sample of the US population. *Br J Nutr*. 2024;131(6):1074–83. doi: 10.1017/S0007114523002568

149 Barabási AL, Menichetti G, Loscalzo J. The unmapped chemical complexity of our diet. *Nat Food*. 2019;1(1):33–7. doi: 10.1038/s43016-019-0005-1

150 Wan Q, Li N, Du L, et al. Allium vegetable consumption and health: an umbrella review of meta-analyses of multiple health outcomes. *Food Sci Nutr*. 2019;7(8):2451–70. doi: 10.1002/fsn3.1117

151 Wise Golden Onion & Garlic Flavored Potato Chips. EWG's Food Scores. Accessed September 28, 2025. https://www.ewg.org/foodscores/products/0041262287488-Wise GoldenOnionGarlicFlavoredPotatoChipsOnionGarlic/

152 Kwon TW, Hong JH, Moon GS, et al. Food technology: challenge for health promotion. *BioFactors*. 2004;22(1–4):279–87. doi: 10.1002/biof.5520220155

153 Lanska DJ. Chapter 30: historical aspects of the major neurological vitamin deficiency disorders: the water-soluble B vitamins. *Handb Clin Neurol*. 2010;95:445–76. doi: 10.1016/S0072-9752(08)02130-1

154 Kwon TW, Hong JH, Moon GS, et al. Food technology: Challenge for health promotion. *BioFactors*. 2004;22(1-4):279–87. doi: 10.1002/biof.5520220155

155 Warner JO. Artificial food additives: hazardous to long-term health? *Arch Dis Child*. 2024;109(11):882–5. doi: 10.1136/archdischild-2023-326565

156 Astrup A, Monteiro CA. Does the concept of "ultra-processed foods" help inform dietary guidelines, beyond conventional classification systems? NO. *Am J Clin Nutr*. 2022;116(6):1482–8. doi: 10.1093/ajcn/nqac123

157 Mambrini SP, Menichetti F, Ravella S, et al. Ultra-processed food consumption and incidence of obesity and cardiometabolic risk factors in adults: a systematic review of prospective studies. *Nutrients*. 2023;15(11):2583. doi: 10.3390/nu15112583

158 Astrup A, Monteiro CA. Does the concept of "ultra-processed foods" help inform dietary guidelines, beyond conventional classification systems? NO. *Am J Clin Nutr*. 2022;116(6):1482–8. doi: 10.1093/ajcn/nqac123

159 Bolhuis DP, Forde CG, Cheng Y, Xu H, Martin N, de Graaf C. Slow food: sustained impact of harder foods on the reduction in energy intake over the course of the day. *PLoS ONE*. 2014;9(4):e93370. doi: 10.1371/journal.pone.0093370

160 de Graaf C, Kok FJ. Slow food, fast food and the control of food intake. *Nat Rev Endocrinol*. 2010;6(5):290–3.

161 Viskaal-van Dongen M, Kok FJ, de Graaf C. Eating rate of commonly consumed foods promotes food and energy intake. *Appetite*. 2011;56(1):25–31. doi: 10.1016/j.appet.2010.11.141

162 Agricultural Research Service, United States Department of Agriculture. Milk, chocolate, fluid, commercial, whole, with added vitamin A and vitamin D. FoodData Central. April 2018. Accessed September 19, 2025. https://fdc.nal.usda.gov/food-details/170879/nutrients

163 Agricultural Research Service, United States Department of Agriculture. Carrots, raw. FoodData Central. April 2018. Accessed September 19, 2025. https://fdc.nal.usda.gov/food-details/2258586/nutrients

164 Forde CG, Mars M, de Graaf K. Ultra-processing or oral processing? A role for energy density and eating rate in moderating energy intake from processed foods. *Curr Dev Nutr*. 2020;4(3):nzaa019. doi: 10.1093/cdn/nzaa01

165 Hall KD, Ayuketah A, Brychta R, et al. Ultra-processed diets cause excess calorie intake and weight gain: an inpatient randomized controlled trial of ad libitum food intake. *Cell Metab.* 2019;30(1):67–77.e3. doi: 10.1016/j.cmet.2019.05.008

166 Hall KD, Ayuketah A, Brychta R, et al. Ultra-processed diets cause excess calorie intake and weight gain: an inpatient randomized controlled trial of ad libitum food intake. *Cell Metab.* 2019;30(1):67–77.e3. doi: 10.1016/j.cmet.2019.05.008

167 Forde CG, Mars M, de Graaf K. Ultra-processing or oral processing? A role for energy density and eating rate in moderating energy intake from processed foods. *Curr Dev Nutr.* 2020;4(3):nzaa019. doi: 10.1093/cdn/nzaa01

168 Agricultural Research Service, United States Department of Agriculture. Oil, olive, salad or cooking. FoodData Central. April 2018. Accessed September 19, 2025. https://fdc.nal.usda.gov/food-details/171413/nutrients

169 Agricultural Research Service, United States Department of Agriculture. Blackberries, raw. FoodData Central. April 2018. Accessed September 28, 2025. https://fdc.nal.usda.gov/food-details/173946/nutrients

170 Agricultural Research Service, United States Department of Agriculture. Cherry tomatoes. FoodData Central. April 2018. Accessed September 28, 2025. https://fdc.nal.usda.gov/food-details/170457/nutrients

171 Agricultural Research Service, United States Department of Agriculture. Jelly Belly, jelly beans. FoodData Central. July 2017. Accessed September 28, 2025. https://fdc.nal.usda.gov/food-details/2047543/nutrients

172 Agricultural Research Service, United States Department of Agriculture. Potatoes, baked, flesh and skin, without salt. FoodData Central. April 2018. Accessed September 28, 2025. https://fdc.nal.usda.gov/food-details/170093/nutrients

173 Agricultural Research Service, United States Department of Agriculture. McDonald's, french fries. FoodData Central. April 2019. Accessed September 28, 2025. https://fdc.nal.usda.gov/food-details/170721/nutrients

174 Gupta S, Hawk T, Aggarwal A, Drewnowski A. Characterizing ultra-processed foods by energy density, nutrient density, and cost. *Front Nutr.* 2019;6:70. doi: 10.3389/fnut.2019.00070

175 Prentice AM, Jebb SA. Fast foods, energy density and obesity: a possible mechanistic link. *Obes Rev.* 2003;4(4):187–94. doi: 10.1046/j.1467-789x.2003.00117.x

176 Prentice AM, Jebb SA. Fast foods, energy density and obesity: a possible mechanistic link. *Obes Rev.* 2003;4(4):187–94. doi: 10.1046/j.1467-789x.2003.00117.x

177 Stender S, Dyerberg J, Astrup A. Fast food: unfriendly and unhealthy. *Int J Obes (Lond).* 2007;31(6):887–90. doi: 10.1038/sj.ijo.0803616

178 Hall KD, Ayuketah A, Brychta R, et al. Ultra-processed diets cause excess calorie intake and weight gain: an inpatient randomized controlled trial of ad libitum food intake. *Cell Metab.* 2019;30(1):67–77.e3. doi: 10.1016/j.cmet.2019.05.008

179 Ledikwe JH, Blanck HM, Khan LK, et al. Dietary energy density determined by eight calculation methods in a nationally representative United States population. *J Nutr.* 2005;135(2):273–8. doi: 10.1093/jn/135.2.273

180 Astrup A, Monteiro CA. Does the concept of "ultra-processed foods" help inform dietary guidelines, beyond conventional classification systems? NO. *Am J Clin Nutr.* 2022;116(6):1482–8. doi: 10.1093/ajcn/nqac123

181 Forde CG, Mars M, de Graaf K. Ultra-processing or oral processing? A role for energy density and eating rate in moderating energy intake from processed foods. *Curr Dev Nutr.* 2020;4(3):nzaa019. doi: 10.1093/cdn/nzaa01.

182 Hall KD, Ayuketah A, Brychta R, et al. Ultra-processed diets cause excess calorie intake and weight gain: an inpatient randomized controlled trial of *ad libitum* food intake. *Cell Metab.* 2019;30(1):67–77.e3. doi: 10.1016/j.cmet.2019.05.008

183 Hall KD, Ayuketah A, Brychta R, et al. Ultra-processed diets cause excess calorie intake and weight gain: an inpatient randomized controlled trial of *ad libitum* food intake. *Cell Metab.* 2019;30(1):67–77.e3. doi: 10.1016/j.cmet.2019.05.008

184 Almy TP. The dietary fiber hypothesis. *Am J Clin Nutr.* 1981;34(3):432–3. doi: 10.1093/ajcn/34.3.432

185 Burkitt DP, Walker AR, Painter NS. Effect of dietary fibre on stools and the transit-times, and its role in the causation of disease. *Lancet.* 1972;2(7792):1408–12. doi: 10.1016/s0140-6736(72)92974-1

186 Moloughney S. Dietary fiber market to reach $3.25 billion by 2017. *Neutraceuticals World.* October 29, 2012. Accessed September 28, 2025. https://nutraceuticalsworld.com/contents/view_breaking-news/2012-10-29/dietary-fiber-market-to-reach-325-billion-by-2017

187 McKeown NM, Fahey GC Jr, Slavin J, van der Kamp JW. Fibre intake for optimal health: how can healthcare professionals support people to reach dietary recommendations?. *BMJ.* 2022;378:e054370. doi:10.1136/bmj-2020-054370

188 Grundy MML, Carrière F, Mackie AR, Gray DA, Butterworth PJ, Ellis PR. The role of plant cell wall encapsulation and porosity in regulating lipolysis during the digestion of almond seeds. *Food Funct.* 2016;7(1):69–78. doi: 10.1039/c5fo00758e

189 Flood-Obbagy JE, Rolls BJ. The effect of fruit in different forms on energy intake and satiety at a meal. *Appetite.* 2009;52(2):416–22. doi: 10.1016/j.appet.2008.12.001

190 Fardet A. A shift toward a new holistic paradigm will help to preserve and better process grain products' food structure for improving their health effects. *Food Funct.* 2015;6(2):363–82. doi: 10.1039/c4fo00477a

191 Capozzi F, Magkos F, Fava F, et al. A multidisciplinary perspective of ultra-processed foods and associated food processing technologies: a view of the sustainable road ahead. *Nutrients.* 2021;13(11):3948. doi: 10.3390/nu13113948

192 Brand J, Nicholson P, Thorburn A, Truswell A. Food processing and the glycemic index. *Am J Clin Nutr.* 1985;42(6):1192–6. doi: 10.1093/ajcn/42.6.1192

193 Atkinson FS, Foster-Powell K, Brand-Miller JC. International tables of glycemic index and glycemic load values: 2008. *Diabetes Care.* 2008;31(12):2281–3. doi: 10.2337/dc08-1239

194 Mackie AR, Bajka BH, Rigby NM, et al. Oatmeal particle size alters glycemic index but not as a function of gastric emptying rate. *Am J Physiol Gastrointest Liver Physiol.* 2017;313(3):G239–46. doi: 10.1152/ajpgi.00005.2017

195   Ludwig DS, Majzoub JA, Al-Zahrani A, Dallal GE, Blanco I, Roberts SB. High glycemic index foods, overeating, and obesity. *Pediatrics*. 1999;103(3):E26. doi: 10.1542/peds.103.3.e26

196   Atkinson FS, Foster-Powell K, Brand-Miller JC. International tables of glycemic index and glycemic load values: 2008. *Diabetes Care*. 2008;31(12):2281–3. doi: 10.2337/dc08-1239

197   Brand JC, Nicholson PL, Thorburn AW, Truswell AS. Food processing and the glycemic index. *Am J Clin Nutr*. 1985;42(6):1192–6. doi: 10.1093/ajcn/42.6.1192

198   Atkinson FS, Foster-Powell K, Brand-Miller JC. International tables of glycemic index and glycemic load values: 2008. *Diabetes Care*. 2008;31(12):2281–3. doi: 10.2337/dc08-1239

199   Wahlqvist ML. Food structure is critical for optimal health. *Food Funct*. 2016;7(3):1245–50. doi: 10.1039/c5fo01285f

200   Willett WC. The dietary pyramid: does the foundation need repair? *Am J Clin Nutr*. 1998;68(2):218–9. doi: 10.1093/ajcn/68.2.218

201   Isaksson H, Rakha A, Andersson R, Fredriksson H, Olsson J, Åman P. Rye kernel breakfast increases satiety in the afternoon – an effect of food structure. *Nutr J*. 2011;10(1):31. doi: 10.1186/1475-2891-10-31

202   Astrup A, Monteiro CA. Does the concept of "ultra-processed foods" help inform dietary guidelines, beyond conventional classification systems? NO. *Am J Clin Nutr*. 2022;116(6):1482–8. doi: 10.1093/ajcn/nqac123

203   Gearhardt AN, DiFeliceantonio AG. Highly processed foods can be considered addictive substances based on established scientific criteria. *Addiction*. 2023;118(4):589–98. doi: 10.1111/add.16065

204   LaFata EM, Allison KC, Audrain-McGovern J, Forman EM. Ultra-processed food addiction: a research update. *Curr Obes Rep*. 2024;13(2):214–23. doi: 10.1007/s13679-024-00569-w

205   LaFata EM, Gearhardt AN. Ultra-processed food addiction: an epidemic? *Psychother Psychosom*. 2022;91(6):363–72. doi: 10.1159/000527322

206   LaFata EM, Gearhardt AN. Ultra-processed food addiction: an epidemic? *Psychother Psychosom*. 2022;91(6):363–72. doi: 10.1159/000527322

207   Fazzino TL, Jun D, Chollet-Hinton L, Bjorlie K. US tobacco companies selectively disseminated hyper-palatable foods into the US food system: empirical evidence and current implications. *Addiction*. 2024;119(1):62–71. doi: 10.1111/add.16332

208   Fazzino TL, Jun D, Chollet-Hinton L, Bjorlie K. US tobacco companies selectively disseminated hyper-palatable foods into the US food system: empirical evidence and current implications. *Addiction*. 2024;119(1):62–71. doi: 10.1111/add.16332

209   Crosbie E, Schmidt L. Commentary on Fazzino *et al* .: proof for why we need cross-industry approaches to research on the commercial determinants of health. *Addiction*. 2024;119(1):72–3. doi: 10.1111/add.16378

210   Fazzino TL, Jun D, Chollet-Hinton L, Bjorlie K. US tobacco companies selectively disseminated hyper-palatable foods into the US food system: empirical evidence and current implications. *Addiction*. 2024;119(1):62–71. doi: 10.1111/add.16332

211 Lustig RH. Ultraprocessed food: addictive, toxic, and ready for regulation. *Nutrients*. 2020;12(11):3401. doi: 10.3390/nu12113401

212 Gearhardt AN, Bueno NB, DiFeliceantonio AG, Roberto CA, Jiménez-Murcia S, Fernandez-Aranda F. Social, clinical, and policy implications of ultra-processed food addiction [published correction appears in *BMJ*. 2023;383:p2679. doi: 10.1136/bmj. p2679.]. *BMJ*. 2023;383:e075354. doi:10.1136/bmj-2023-075354

213 Schulte EM, Avena NM, Gearhardt AN. Which foods may be addictive? The roles of processing, fat content, and glycemic load. *PLoS ONE*. 2015;10(2):e0117959. doi: 10.1371/journal.pone.0117959

214 Nestle M. Regulating the food industry: an aspirational agenda. *Am J Public Health*. 2022;112(6):853–8. doi: 10.2105/AJPH.2022.306844

215 LaFata EM, Allison KC, Audrain-McGovern J, Forman EM. Ultra-processed food addiction: a research update. *Curr Obes Rep*. 2024;13(2):214–23. doi: 10.1007/s13679-024-00569-w

216 Gearhardt AN, Bueno NB, DiFeliceantonio AG, Roberto CA, Jiménez-Murcia S, Fernandez-Aranda F. Social, clinical, and policy implications of ultra-processed food addiction. *BMJ*. 2023;383:e075354. doi:10.1136/bmj-2023-075354

217 Schulte EM, Avena NM, Gearhardt AN. Which foods may be addictive? The roles of processing, fat content, and glycemic load. *PLoS ONE*. 2015;10(2):e0117959.

218 Meule A. Back by popular demand: a narrative review on the history of food addiction research. *Yale J Biol Med*. 2015;88(3):295–302.

219 Lenoir M, Serre F, Cantin L, Ahmed SH. Intense sweetness surpasses cocaine reward. *PLoS ONE*. 2007;2(8):e698.

220 Dillehay TD, Rossen J, Ugent D, Karathanasis A, Vásquez V, Netherly P. Early Holocene coca chewing in northern Peru. *Antiquity*. 2010;84(326):939–53.

221 Weil AT. Coca leaf as a therapeutic agent. *Am J Drug Alcohol Abuse*. 1978;5(1):75–86. doi: 10.3109/00952997809029262

222 Verebey K, Gold MS. From coca leaves to crack: the effects of dose and routes of administration in abuse liability. *Psychiatric Annals*. 1988;18(9):513–20. doi:10.3928/0048-5713-19880901-06

223 Ifland J, Preuss HG, Marcus MT, Rourke KM, Taylor W, Wright HT. Clearing the confusion around processed food addiction. *J Am Coll Nutr*. 2015;34(3):240–3. doi: 10.1080/07315724.2015.1022466

224 Belkova J, Rozkot M, Danek P, Klein P, Matonohova J, Podhorna I. Sugar and nutritional extremism. *Crit Rev Food Sci Nutr*. 2017;57(5):933–6. doi: 10.1080/10408398.2014.940027

225 Lustig RH. Ultraprocessed food: addictive, toxic, and ready for regulation. *Nutrients*. 2020;12(11):3401. doi: 10.3390/nu12113401

226 Volkow ND, Wang GJ, Tomasi D, Baler RD. Obesity and addiction: neurobiological overlaps. *Obes Rev*. 2013;14(1):2–18. doi: 10.1111/j.1467-789X.2012.01031.x

227 Volkow ND, Wang GJ, Baler RD. Reward, dopamine and the control of food intake: implications for obesity. *Trends Cogn Sci*. 2011;15(1):37–46. doi: 10.1016/j.tics.2010.11.001

228 Ott V, Finlayson G, Lehnert H, et al. Oxytocin reduces reward-driven food intake in humans. *Diabetes*. 2013;62(10):3418–25. doi: 10.2337/db13-0663

229 Small DM, Jones-Gotman M, Dagher A. Feeding-induced dopamine release in dorsal striatum correlates with meal pleasantness ratings in healthy human volunteers. *Neuroimage*. 2003;19(4):1709–15. doi: 10.1016/s1053-8119(03)00253-2

230 Szczypka MS, Kwok K, Brot MD, et al. Dopamine production in the caudate putamen restores feeding in dopamine-deficient mice. *Neuron*. 2001;30(3):819–28. doi: 10.1016/s0896-6273(01)00319-1

231 LaFata EM, Gearhardt AN. Ultra-processed food addiction: an epidemic? *Psychother Psychosom*. 2022;91(6):363–72. doi: 10.1159/000527322

232 Janssen HG, Davies IG, Richardson LD, Stevenson L. Determinants of takeaway and fast food consumption: a narrative review. *Nutr Res Rev*. 2018;31(1):16–34. doi: 10.1017/S0954422417000178

233 Crosbie E, Schmidt L. Commentary on Fazzino *et al*.: proof for why we need cross-industry approaches to research on the commercial determinants of health. *Addiction*. 2024;119(1):72–3. doi: 10.1111/add.16378

234 Gearhardt AN, Bueno NB, DiFeliceantonio AG, Roberto CA, Jiménez-Murcia S, Fernandez-Aranda F. Social, clinical, and policy implications of ultra-processed food addiction [published correction appears in *BMJ*. 2023;383:p2679. doi: 10.1136/bmj.p2679.]. *BMJ*. 2023;383:e075354. doi:10.1136/bmj-2023-075354

235 Gearhardt AN, DiFeliceantonio AG. Highly processed foods can be considered addictive substances based on established scientific criteria. *Addiction*. 2023;118(4):589–98. doi: 10.1111/add.16065

236 Gearhardt AN, DiFeliceantonio AG. Highly processed foods can be considered addictive substances based on established scientific criteria. *Addiction*. 2023;118(4):589–98. doi: 10.1111/add.16065

237 Harrison D, Bueno M, Yamada J, Adams-Webber T, Stevens B. Analgesic effects of sweet-tasting solutions for infants: current state of equipoise. *Pediatrics*. 2010;126(5):894–902. doi: 10.1542/peds.2010-1593

238 Trenchard E, Silverstone T. Naloxone reduces the food intake of normal human volunteers. *Appetite*. 1983;4(1):43–50. doi: 10.1016/s0195-6663(83)80045-2.

239 Gearhardt AN, DiFeliceantonio AG. Highly processed foods can be considered addictive substances based on established scientific criteria. *Addiction*. 2023;118(4):589–98. doi: 10.1111/add.16065

240 Gearhardt AN, DiFeliceantonio AG. Highly processed foods can be considered addictive substances based on established scientific criteria. *Addiction*. 2023;118(4):589–98. doi: 10.1111/add.16065

241 LaFata EM, Allison KC, Audrain-McGovern J, Forman EM. Ultra-processed food addiction: a research update. *Curr Obes Rep*. 2024;13(2):214–23. doi: 10.1007/s13679-024-00569-w

242 Hu S, Gearhardt AN, LaFata EM. Development of the modified highly processed food withdrawal scale (mProWS). *Appetite*. 2024;198:107370. doi: 10.1016/j.appet.2024.107370

243 Avena NM, Rada P, Hoebel BG. Evidence for sugar addiction: behavioral and neurochemical effects of intermittent, excessive sugar intake. *Neurosci Biobehav Rev.* 2008;32(1):20–39. doi: 10.1016/j.neubiorev.2007.04.019

244 Burger KS, Stice E. Frequent ice cream consumption is associated with reduced striatal response to receipt of an ice cream–based milkshake. *Am J Clin Nutr.* 2012;95(4):810–7. doi: 10.3945/ajcn.111.027003

245 Wiss DA, LaFata EM. Ultra-processed foods and mental health: where do eating disorders fit into the puzzle? *Nutrients.* 2024;16(12):1955. doi: 10.3390/nu16121955

246 Ifland J, Preuss HG, Marcus MT, Rourke KM, Taylor W, Wright HT. Clearing the confusion around processed food addiction. *J Am Coll Nutr.* 2015;34(3):240–3. doi: 10.1080/07315724.2015.1022466.

247 Gearhardt AN, Schulte EM. Is food addictive? A review of the science. *Annu Rev Nutr.* 2021;41(1):387–410. doi: 10.1146/annurev-nutr-110420-111710

248 Anthony JC, Warner LA, Kessler RC. Comparative epidemiology of dependence on tobacco, alcohol, controlled substances, and inhalants: basic findings from the National Comorbidity Survey. *Exp Clin Psychopharmacol.* 1994;2(3):244–68. doi: 10.1037/1064-1297.2.3.244

249 Rogers PJ. Food and drug addictions: similarities and differences. *Pharmacol Biochem Behav.* 2017;153:182–90. doi: 10.1016/j.pbb.2017.01.001

250 Robinson JH, Pritchard WS. The meaning of addiction: reply to West. *Psychopharmacol.* 1992;108(4):411–6. doi: 10.1007/BF02247414

251 Rogers PJ. Food and drug addictions: similarities and differences. *Pharmacol Biochem Behav.* 2017;153:182–90. doi: 10.1016/j.pbb.2017.01.001

252 Kaplan R. Carrot addiction. *Aust N Z J Psychiatry.* 1996;30(5):698–700. doi: 10.3109/00048679609062670

253 Ayton A, Ibrahim A, Dugan J, Galvin E, Wright OW. Ultra-processed foods and binge eating: a retrospective observational study. *Nutrition.* 2021;84:111023. doi: 10.1016/j. nut.2020.111023

254 Monteiro CA, Cannon G, Moubarac JC, Levy RB, Louzada MLC, Jaime PC. The UN Decade of Nutrition, the NOVA food classification and the trouble with ultra-processing. *Public Health Nutr.* 2018;21(1):5–17. doi: 10.1017/S1368980017000234

255 Monteiro CA. Nutrition and health. The issue is not food, nor nutrients, so much as processing. *Public Health Nutr.* 2009;12(5):729–31. doi: 10.1017/S1368980009005291

256 Lawrence M. Ultra-processed foods: a fit-for-purpose concept for nutrition policy activities to tackle unhealthy and unsustainable diets. *Br J Nutr.* 2023;129(12):2195–8. doi: 10.1017/S0007114523000016.

257 Scrinis G. Reformulation, fortification and functionalization: Big Food corporations' nutritional engineering and marketing strategies. *J Peasant Stud.* 2016;43(1):17–37. doi: 10.1080/03066150.2015.1101455

258 Braesco V, Souchon I, Sauvant P, et al. Ultra-processed foods: how functional is the NOVA system? *Eur J Clin Nutr.* 2022;76(9):1245–53. doi: 10.1038/s41430-022-01099-1

259 *Jacobellis v. Ohio*, 378 US 184 (1964).

260 Braesco V, Souchon I, Sauvant P, et al. Ultra-processed foods: how functional is the NOVA system? *Eur J Clin Nutr*. 2022;76(9):1245–53. doi: 10.1038/s41430-022-01099-1

261 Lawrence M. Ultra-processed foods: a fit-for-purpose concept for nutrition policy activities to tackle unhealthy and unsustainable diets. *Br J Nutr*. 2023;129(12):2195–8. doi: 10.1017/S0007114523000016

262 Medina-Meza IG, Vaidya Y, Barnaba C. FooDOxS: a database of oxidized sterols content in foods. *Food Funct*. 2024;15(12):6324–34. doi: 10.1039/d4fo00678j

263 Lawrence M. Ultra-processed foods: a fit-for-purpose concept for nutrition policy activities to tackle unhealthy and unsustainable diets. *Br J Nutr*. 2023;129(12):2195–8. doi: 10.1017/S0007114523000016

264 Astrup A, Monteiro CA. Does the concept of "ultra-processed foods" help inform dietary guidelines, beyond conventional classification systems? Debate consensus. *Am J Clin Nutr*. 2022;116(6):1489–91. doi: 10.1093/ajcn/nqac230

265 Sanchez-Siles L, Roman S, Fogliano V, Siegrist M. Naturalness and healthiness in "ultra-processed foods": a multidisciplinary perspective and case study. *Trends Food Sci Technol*. 2022;129:667–73. doi: 10.1016/j.tifs.2022.11.009

266 Levine AS, Ubbink J. Ultra-processed foods: processing versus formulation. *Obes Sci Pract*. 2023;9(4):435–9. doi: 10.1002/osp4.657

267 Knorr D. Food processing: legacy, significance and challenges. *Trends Food Sci Technol*. 2024;143:104270. doi: 10.1016/j.tifs.2023.104270

268 Monteiro CA, Cannon G, Lawrence M, Costa Louzada ML, Pereira Machado P. *Ultra-processed Foods, Diet Quality, and Health Using the NOVA Classification System*. Food and Agriculture Organization of the United Nations; 2019. Accessed April 24, 2025. https://openknowledge.fao.org/server/api/core/bitstreams/5277b379-0acb-4d97-a6a3-602774104629/content

269 Monteiro CA. Nutrition and health. The issue is not food, nor nutrients, so much as processing. *Public Health Nutr*. 2009;12(5):729–31. doi: 10.1017/S1368980009005291

270 Vitale M, Costabile G, Testa R, et al. Ultra-processed foods and human health: a systematic review and meta-analysis of prospective cohort studies. *Adv Nutr*. 2024;15(1):100121. doi: 10.1016/j.advnut.2023.09.009

271 Jones JM. Food processing: criteria for dietary guidance and public health? *Proc Nutr Soc*. 2019;78(1):4–18. doi: 10.1017/S0029665118002513

272 Lawrence M. Ultra-processed foods: a fit-for-purpose concept for nutrition policy activities to tackle unhealthy and unsustainable diets. *Br J Nutr*. 2023;129(12):2195–8. doi: 10.1017/S0007114523000016

273 Kelly OJ. Ultraprocessed food is not a replacement for whole food. *Adv Nutr*. 2023;14(5):1244–5. doi: 10.1016/j.advnut.2023.05.016

274 Arnold D. British India and the "beriberi problem", 1798–1942. *Med Hist*. 2010;54(3):295–314. doi: 10.1017/s0025727300004622

275 Bollet AJ. Politics and pellagra: the epidemic of pellagra in the U.S. in the early twentieth century. *Yale J Biol Med*. 1992;65(3):211–21. PMID: 1285449

276 Kirkland JB, Meyer-Ficca ML. Niacin. In: *Advances in Food and Nutrition Research*. Vol 83. Elsevier; 2018:83–149. doi: 10.1016/bs.afnr.2017.11.003

277 Vadiveloo MK, Gardner CD. Not all ultra-processed foods are created equal: a case for advancing research and policy that balances health and nutrition security. *Diabetes Care*. 2023;46(7):1327–9. doi: 10.2337/dci23-0018

278 Cummings KM, Brown A, O'Connor R. The cigarette controversy. *Cancer Epidemiol Biomarkers Prev*. 2007;16(6):1070–6. doi: 10.1158/1055-9965.EPI-06-0912

279 Kelly OJ. Ultraprocessed food is not a replacement for whole food. *Adv Nutr*. 2023;14(5):1244–5. doi: 10.1016/j.advnut.2023.05.016

280 Sanchez-Siles L, Roman S, Fogliano V, Siegrist M. Naturalness and healthiness in "ultra-processed foods": a multidisciplinary perspective and case study. *Trends Food Sci Technol*. 2022;129:667–73. doi: 10.1016/j.tifs.2022.11.009

281 Chen A, Kayrala N, Trapeau M, Aoun M, Bordenave N. The clean label trend: an ineffective heuristic that disserves both consumers and the food industry? *Comp Rev Food Sci Food Safe*. 2022;21(6):4921–38. doi: 10.1111/1541-4337.13031

282 Gibney MJ. Ultra-processed foods: definitions and policy issues. *Curr Dev Nutr*. 2019;3(2):nzy077. doi: 10.1093/cdn/nzy077

283 Braesco V, Souchon I, Sauvant P, et al. Ultra-processed foods: how functional is the NOVA system? *Eur J Clin Nutr*. 2022;76(9):1245–53. doi: 10.1038/s41430-022-01099-1

284 Capozzi F, Magkos F, Fava F, et al. A multidisciplinary perspective of ultra-processed foods and associated food processing technologies: a view of the sustainable road ahead. *Nutrients*. 2021;13(11):3948. doi: 10.3390/nu13113948

285 Visioli F, Marangoni F, Fogliano V, et al. The ultra-processed foods hypothesis: a product processed well beyond the basic ingredients in the package. *Nutr Res Rev*. 2023;36(2):340–50. doi: 10.1017/S0954422422000117

286 Morales-Berstein F, Biessy C, Viallon V, et al. Ultra-processed foods, adiposity and risk of head and neck cancer and oesophageal adenocarcinoma in the European Prospective Investigation into Cancer and Nutrition study: a mediation analysis. *Eur J Nutr*. 2024;63(2):377–96. doi: 10.1007/s00394-023-03270-1

287 Morales-Berstein F, Biessy C, Viallon V, et al. Ultra-processed foods, adiposity and risk of head and neck cancer and oesophageal adenocarcinoma in the European Prospective Investigation into Cancer and Nutrition study: a mediation analysis. *Eur J Nutr*. 2024;63(2):377–96. doi: 10.1007/s00394-023-03270-1

288 Barbaresko J, Bröder J, Conrad J, Szczerba E, Lang A, Schlesinger S. Ultra-processed food consumption and human health: an umbrella review of systematic reviews with meta-analyses. *Crit Rev Food Sci Nutr*. 2025;65(11):1999–2007. doi: 10.1080/10408398.2024.2317877

289 Sherling DH, Hennekens CH, Ferris AH. Newest updates to health providers on the hazards of ultra-processed foods and proposed solutions. *Am J Med*. 2024;137(5):395–8. doi: 10.1016/j.amjmed.2024.02.001

290 Adams J, Hofman K, Moubarac JC, Thow AM. Public health response to ultra-processed food and drinks. *BMJ*. 2020;369:m2391. doi: 10.1136/bmj.m2391

291 Sherling DH, Hennekens CH, Ferris AH. Newest updates to health providers on the hazards of ultra-processed foods and proposed solutions. *Am J Med*. 2024;137(5):395–8. doi: 10.1016/j.amjmed.2024.02.001

292 Logan AC, D'Adamo CR, Pizzorno JE, Prescott SL. "Food faddists and pseudoscientists!": reflections on the history of resistance to ultra-processed foods. *EXPLORE*. 2024;20(4):470–6. doi: 10.1016/j.explore.2023.12.014

293 Logan AC, D'Adamo CR, Pizzorno JE, Prescott SL. "Food faddists and pseudoscientists!": reflections on the history of resistance to ultra-processed foods. *EXPLORE*. 2024;20(4):470–6. doi: 10.1016/j.explore.2023.12.014

294 Logan AC, D'Adamo CR, Pizzorno JE, Prescott SL. "Food faddists and pseudoscientists!": reflections on the history of resistance to ultra-processed foods. *EXPLORE*. 2024;20(4):470–6. doi: 10.1016/j.explore.2023.12.014

295 Popkin BM, Armstrong LE, Bray GA, Caballero B, Frei B, Willett WC. Reply to RJ Kaplan. *Am J Clin Nutr*. 2006;84(5):1249–51. doi: 10.1093/ajcn/84.5.1249

296 Logan AC, D'Adamo CR, Pizzorno JE, Prescott SL. "Food faddists and pseudoscientists!": reflections on the history of resistance to ultra-processed foods. *EXPLORE*. 2024;20(4):470–6. doi: 10.1016/j.explore.2023.12.014

297 Carriedo A, Pinsky I, Crosbie E, Ruskin G, Mialon M. The corporate capture of the nutrition profession in the USA: the case of the Academy of Nutrition and Dietetics. *Public Health Nutr*. 2022;25(12):3568–82. doi: 10.1017/S1368980022001835

298 Popkin BM, Armstrong LE, Bray GA, Caballero B, Frei B, Willett WC. Reply to RJ Kaplan. *Am J Clin Nutr*. 2006;84(5):1249–51. doi: 10.1093/ajcn/84.5.1249

299 "All foods fit.": dietitians give their top tips for better nutrition. Orlando Health. September 23, 2024. Accessed April 16, 2025. https://www.orlandohealth.com/content-hub/all-foods-fit-dietitians-give-their-top-tips-for-better-nutrition

300 Logan AC, D'Adamo CR, Pizzorno JE, Prescott SL. "Food faddists and pseudoscientists!": reflections on the history of resistance to ultra-processed foods. *EXPLORE*. 2024;20(4):470–6. doi: 10.1016/j.explore.2023.12.014

301 Popkin BM, Armstrong LE, Bray GA, Caballero B, Frei B, Willett WC. Reply to RJ Kaplan. *Am J Clin Nutr*. 2006;84(5):1249–51. doi: 10.1093/ajcn/84.5.1249

302 Chopra M, Darnton-Hill I. Tobacco and obesity epidemics: not so different after all? *BMJ*. 2004;328(7455):1558–60. doi: 10.1136/bmj.328.7455.1558

303 Lauber K, McGee D, Gilmore AB. Commercial use of evidence in public health policy: a critical assessment of food industry submissions to global-level consultations on non-communicable disease prevention. *BMJ Glob Health*. 2021;6(8). doi: 10.1136/bmjgh-2021-006176

304 Gómez EJ, Maani N, Galea S. The pitfalls of ascribing moral agency to corporations: public obligation and political and social contexts in the commercial determinants of health. *Milbank Q*. 2024;102(1):28–42. doi: 10.1111/1468-0009.12678

305 Chung H, Cullerton K, Lacy-Nichols J. Mapping the lobbying footprint of harmful industries: 23 years of data from opensecrets. *Milbank Q*. 2024;102(1):212–32. doi: 10.1111/1468-0009.12686

306 Monteiro CA. Nutrition and health. The issue is not food, nor nutrients, so much as processing. *Public Health Nutr*. 2009;12(5):729–31. doi: 10.1017/S1368980009005291

307 Popkin BM. Agricultural policies, food and public health. *EMBO Rep*. 2011;12(1):11–8. doi: 10.1038/embor.2010.200

308 Visioli F, Marangoni F, Fogliano V, et al. The ultra-processed foods hypothesis: a product processed well beyond the basic ingredients in the package. *Nutr Res Rev.* 2023;36(2):340–50. doi: 10.1017/S0954422422000117

309 LaFata EM, Gearhardt AN. Ultra-processed food addiction: an epidemic? *Psychother Psychosom.* 2022;91(6):363–72. doi: 10.1159/000527322

310 Wood B, Robinson E, Baker P, et al. What is the purpose of ultra-processed food? An exploratory analysis of the financialisation of ultra-processed food corporations and implications for public health. *Global Health.* 2023;19(1):85. doi: 10.1186/s12992-023-00990-1

311 Lustig RH. Ultraprocessed food: addictive, toxic, and ready for regulation. *Nutrients.* 2020;12(11):3401. doi: 10.3390/nu12113401

312 Cohen DA, Lesser LI. Obesity prevention at the point of purchase. *Obes Rev.* 2016;17(5):389–96. doi: 10.1111/obr.12387

313 Neal B. Fat chance for physical activity. *Popul Health Metrics.* 2013;11(1):9. doi: 10.1186/1478-7954-11-9

314 Lawrence MA, Baker PI. Ultra-processed food and adverse health outcomes. *BMJ.* 2019;365:l2289. doi: 10.1136/bmj.l2289

315 Lustig RH. Ethical considerations for nutrition counseling about processed food—reply. *JAMA Pediatr.* 2017;171(9):914. doi: 10.1001/jamapediatrics.2017.1906

316 LaFata EM, Allison KC, Audrain-McGovern J, Forman EM. Ultra-processed food addiction: a research update. *Curr Obes Rep.* 2024;13(2):214–23. doi: 10.1007/s13679-024-00569-w

317 Pomeranz JL, Mande JR, Mozaffarian D. U.S. policies addressing ultraprocessed foods, 1980–2022. *Am J Prev Med.* 2023;65(6):1134–41. doi: 10.1016/j.amepre.2023.07.006

318 Thomas C, Breeze P, Cummins S, Cornelsen L, Yau A, Brennan A. The health, cost and equity impacts of restrictions on the advertisement of high fat, salt and sugar products across the transport for London network: a health economic modelling study. *Int J Behav Nutr Phys Act.* 2022;19(1):93. doi: 10.1186/s12966-022-01331-y

319 Anderson GK. The addition of synthetic vitamins to confectionery. JAMA. 1945;127(6):331. doi:10.1001/jama.1945.02860060029009

320 Trix Loaded family size breakfast cereal. Nutritionix. Accessed April 21, 2025. https://www.nutritionix.com/i/trix/cereal-loaded-family-size/656058fb9dc25c0008f8f8b9

321 Froot Loops with Marshmallows family size breakfast cereal. Nutritionix. Accessed April 21, 2025. https://www.nutritionix.com/i/froot-loops/cereal-with-marshmallows-family-size/62ea55c2757a2d0008b8218e

322 Stanton RA. Changing eating patterns versus adding nutrients to processed foods. *Med J Aust.* 2016;204(11):398. doi: 10.5694/mja16.00094

323 Cereal boxes, Marshmallow Pebbles, Bedrock Dinosaur Safari (2010). Cereal.Fandom.com. Accessed October 2, 2025. https://cereal.fandom.com/wiki/Cereal_Boxes_-_Marshmallow_Pebbles_-_Bedrock_Dinosaur_Safari_(2010)

324 Lacy-Nichols J, Hattersley L, Scrinis G. Nutritional marketing of plant-based meat-analogue products: an exploratory study of front-of-pack and website claims in the USA. *Public Health Nutr.* 2021;24(14):4430–41. doi: 10.1017/S1368980021002792

325 Monteiro CA, Cannon G. Commentary. The food system. Product reformulation will not improve public health. *World Nutr.* 2012;3(9):406–34.

326 Scrinis G, Monteiro CA. Ultra-processed foods and the limits of product reformulation. *Public Health Nutr.* 2018;21(1):247–52. doi: 10.1017/S1368980017001392

327 Campbell N, Browne S, Claudy M, Reilly K, Finucane FM. Ultra-processed food: the tragedy of the biological commons. *Int J Health Policy Manag.* 2023;12:7557. doi: 10.34172/ijhpm.2022.7557

328 Scott C, Nixon L. The shift in framing of food and beverage product reformulation in the United States from 1980 to 2015. *Crit Public Health.* 2018;28(5):606–18. doi: 10.1080/09581596.2017.1332756

329 Lorillard advertisement for True cigarettes. Stanford University. Accessed April 22, 2025. https://tobacco.stanford.edu/cigarette/img3294/

330 Monteiro CA, Cannon G. Commentary. The food system. Product reformulation will not improve public health. *World Nutr.* 2012;3(9):406–34.

331 Scrinis G. Reformulation, fortification and functionalization: Big Food corporations' nutritional engineering and marketing strategies. *J Peasant Stud.* 2016;43(1):17–37. doi: 10.1080/03066150.2015.1101455

332 Monteiro CA, Cannon G, Moubarac JC, Levy RB, Louzada MLC, Jaime PC. The UN Decade of Nutrition, the NOVA food classification and the trouble with ultra-processing. *Public Health Nutr.* 2018;21(1):5–17. doi: 10.1017/S1368980017000234

333 Assaf S, Park J, Chowdhry N, et al. Unraveling the evolutionary diet mismatch and its contribution to the deterioration of body composition. *Metabolites.* 2024;14(7):379. doi: 10.3390/metabo14070379

334 Trumbo PR, Bleiweiss-Sande R, Campbell JK, et al. Toward a science-based classification of processed foods to support meaningful research and effective health policies. *Front Nutr.* 2024;11:1389601. doi: 10.3389/fnut.2024.1389601

335 Touvier M, da Costa Louzada ML, Mozaffarian D, Baker P, Juul F, Srour B. Ultra-processed foods and cardiometabolic health: public health policies to reduce consumption cannot wait. *BMJ.* 2023;383:e075294. doi: 10.1136/bmj-2023-075294

336 Scrinis G, Monteiro CA. Ultra-processed foods and the limits of product reformulation. *Public Health Nutr.* 2018;21(1):247–52. doi: 10.1017/S1368980017001392

337 Five billion people unprotected from trans fat leading to heart disease. *Neurosciences* (Riyadh). 2023;28(2):155–6. PMID: 37045453

338 LaFata EM, Gearhardt AN. Ultra-processed food addiction: an epidemic? *Psychother Psychosom.* 2022;91(6):363–72. doi: 10.1159/000527322

339 Cadham CJ, Sanchez-Romero LM, Fleischer NL, et al. The actual and anticipated effects of a menthol cigarette ban: a scoping review. *BMC Public Health.* 2020;20(1):1055. doi:10.1186/s12889-020-09055-z

340 Keast RSJ, Swinburn BA, Sayompark D, Whitelock S, Riddell LJ. Caffeine increases sugar-sweetened beverage consumption in a free-living population: a randomised controlled trial. *Br J Nutr.* 2015;113(2):366–371. doi: 10.1017/S000711451400378X

341 Sun H, Liu Y, Xu Y, et al. Global disease burden attributed to high sugar-sweetened beverages in 204 countries and territories from 1990 to 2019. *Prev Med.* 2023;175:107690. doi: 10.1016/j.ypmed.2023.107690

342 Keast RSJ, Swinburn BA, Sayompark D, Whitelock S, Riddell LJ. Caffeine increases sugar-sweetened beverage consumption in a free-living population: a randomised controlled trial. *Br J Nutr.* 2015;113(2):366–71. doi: 10.1017/S000711451400378X

343 Mozaffarian D, El-Abbadi NH, O'Hearn M, et al. Food Compass is a nutrient profiling system using expanded characteristics for assessing healthfulness of foods. *Nat Food.* 2021;2(10):809–18. doi: 10.1038/s43016-021-00381-y.

344 O'Hearn M, Erndt-Marino J, Gerber S, et al. Validation of Food Compass with a healthy diet, cardiometabolic health, and mortality among U.S. adults, 1999–2018. *Nat Commun.* 2022;13(1):7066. doi: 10.1038/s41467-022-34195-8

345 Mozaffarian D, El-Abbadi NH, O'Hearn M, et al. Food Compass is a nutrient profiling system using expanded characteristics for assessing healthfulness of foods. *Nat Food.* 2021;2(10):809–18. doi: 10.1038/s43016-021-00381-y.

346 O'Hearn M, Erndt-Marino J, Gerber S, et al. Validation of Food Compass with a healthy diet, cardiometabolic health, and mortality among U.S. adults, 1999–2018. *Nat Commun.* 2022;13(1):7066. doi: 10.1038/s41467-022-34195-8

347 Mozaffarian D, El-Abbadi NH, O'Hearn M, et al. Food Compass is a nutrient profiling system using expanded characteristics for assessing healthfulness of foods. *Nat Food.* 2021;2(10):809–18. doi: 10.1038/s43016-021-00381-y.

348 Monteiro CA, Cannon G, Moubarac JC, Levy RB, Louzada MLC, Jaime PC. Ultra-processing. An odd 'appraisal.' *Public Health Nutr.* 2018;21(03):497–501. doi: 10.1017/S1368980017003287

349 Mozaffarian D, El-Abbadi NH, O'Hearn M, et al. Food Compass is a nutrient profiling system using expanded characteristics for assessing healthfulness of foods. *Nat Food.* 2021;2(10):809–18. doi: 10.1038/s43016-021-00381-y

350 Mozaffarian D, El-Abbadi NH, O'Hearn M, et al. Food Compass is a nutrient profiling system using expanded characteristics for assessing healthfulness of foods. *Nat Food.* 2021;2(10):809–18. doi: 10.1038/s43016-021-00381-y

351 Dai S, Wellens J, Yang N, et al. Ultra-processed foods and human health: an umbrella review and updated meta-analyses of observational evidence. *Clin Nutr.* 2024;43(6):1386–94. doi: 10.1016/j.clnu.2024.04.016

352 Lichtenstein AH, Appel LJ, Vadiveloo M, et al. 2021 dietary guidance to improve cardiovascular health: a scientific statement from the American Heart Association. *Circulation.* 2021;144(23). doi: 10.1161/CIR.0000000000001031

353 Bradbury KE, Mackay S. Ultra-processed foods linked to higher mortality. *BMJ.* 2024;385. doi: 10.1136/bmj.q793

354 Islami F, Nargis N, Liu Q, et al. Averted lung cancer deaths due to reductions in cigarette smoking in the United States, 1970-2022. *CA Cancer J Clin.* 2025;75(3):216–25. doi: 10.3322/caac.70005

355 Surveillance, Epidemiology, and End Results Program. Cancer stat facts: common cancer sites. National Cancer Institute. Accessed October 15, 2025. https://seer.cancer.gov/statfacts/html/common.html

356 Huang Y, Cao D, Chen Z, et al. Red and processed meat consumption and cancer outcomes: umbrella review. *Food Chem*. 2021;356:129697. doi: 10.1016/j.foodchem.2021.129697

357 Zhang X, Liang S, Chen X, et al. Red/processed meat consumption and non-cancer-related outcomes in humans: umbrella review. *Br J Nutr*. 2023;130(3):484–94. doi: 10.1017/S0007114522003415

358 Lichtenstein AH, Appel LJ, Vadiveloo M, et al. 2021 dietary guidance to improve cardiovascular health: a scientific statement from the American Heart Association. *Circulation*. 2021;144(23). doi: 10.1161/CIR.0000000000001031

359 Mozaffarian D, El-Abbadi NH, O'Hearn M, et al. Food Compass is a nutrient profiling system using expanded characteristics for assessing healthfulness of foods. *Nat Food*. 2021;2(10):809–18. doi: 10.1038/s43016-021-00381-y

360 Visioli F, Marangoni F, Fogliano V, et al. The ultra-processed foods hypothesis: a product processed well beyond the basic ingredients in the package. *Nutr Res Rev*. 2023;36(2):340–50. doi: 10.1017/S0954422422000117

361 KitKat cereal. Nestlé Cereals. Accessed April 22, 2025. https://www.nestle-cereals.com/global/cereals/kitkat

362 KitKat Chocolatey Cereal, breakfast cereal made with whole grain, 11.5 oz . Walmart.com. Accessed October 3, 2025. https://www.walmart.com/ip/KIT-KAT-Chocolatey-Cereal-Breakfast-Cereal-Made-with-Whole-Grain-11-5-oz/2431761399

363 Yeo GSH. Breaking our daily "ultra-processed" bread. *PLoS Med*. 2024;21(7):e1004437. doi: 10.1371/journal.pmed.1004437

364 Augustin LSA, D'Angelo A, Palumbo E, La Vecchia C. Ultraprocessed foods and cancer risk: the importance of distinguishing ultraprocessed food groups. *Eur J Cancer Prev*. 2025;34(2):97–9. doi: 10.1097/CEJ.0000000000000901

365 Bradbury KE, Mackay S. Ultra-processed foods linked to higher mortality. *BMJ*. 2024;385. doi: 10.1136/bmj.q793

366 National Cancer Institute. *Identification of Top Food Sources of Various Dietary Components*. Epidemiology and Genomics Research Program; 2010. Updated November 30, 2019. Accessed April 16, 2025. https://epi.grants.cancer.gov/diet/foodsources

367 GBD 2017 Diet Collaborators. Health effects of dietary risks in 195 countries, 1990-2017: a systematic analysis for the Global Burden of Disease Study 2017 [published correction appears in Lancet. 2021 Jun 26;397(10293):2466. doi: 10.1016/S0140-6736(21)01342-8.]. *Lancet*. 2019;393(10184):1958–72. doi:10.1016/S0140-6736(19)30041-8

368 Hess JM, Comeau ME, Casperson S, et al. Dietary guidelines meet NOVA: developing a menu for a healthy dietary pattern using ultra-processed foods. *J Nutr*. 2023;153(8):2472–81. doi: 10.1016/j.tjnut.2023.06.028

369 Stall S. Bread has salt: options for very low-sodium bread. *J Ren Nutr*. 2013;23(1):e5–9. doi: 10.1053/j.jrn.2012.10.005

370 Mighty Manna whole rye bread. Manna Organics. Accessed April 22, 2025. https://mannaorganicbakery.com/product/sprouted-whole-rye-organic-bread/

371 Vargas MCA, Simsek S. Clean label in bread. *Foods*. 2021;10(9):2054. doi: 10.3390/foods10092054

372 Shanmugavel V, Komala Santhi K, Kurup AH, Kalakandan S, Anandharaj A, Rawson A. Potassium bromate: effects on bread components, health, environment and method of analysis: a review. *Food Chem*. 2020;311:125964. doi: 10.1016/j.foodchem.2019.125964

373 Liang Z, Gao J, Yu P, Yang D. History, mechanism of action, and toxicity: a review of commonly used dough rheology improvers. *Crit Rev Food Sci Nutr*. 2023;63(7):947–63. doi: 10.1080/10408398.2021.1956427

374 California Food Safety Act, AB No 418, ch 328 (Ca 2023).

375 Vitale M, Costabile G, Testa R, et al. Ultra-processed foods and human health: a systematic review and meta-analysis of prospective cohort studies. *Adv Nutr*. 2024;15(1):100121. doi: 10.1016/j.advnut.2023.09.009

376 Mozaffarian D, El-Abbadi NH, O'Hearn M, et al. Food Compass is a nutrient profiling system using expanded characteristics for assessing healthfulness of foods. *Nat Food*. 2021;2(10):809–18. doi: 10.1038/s43016-021-00381-y

377 Uncle Sam Original cereal. EWG. Accessed April 22, 2025. https://www.ewg.org/foodscores/products/041653456783-UncleSamOriginalWheatBerryFlakes/

378 Hunt's Tomato Sauce. Hunt's. Accessed April 22, 2025. https://www.hunts.com/tomato-sauce-and-paste/tomato-sauce

379 Ragu Simply Traditional Sauce. Ragu. Accessed April 22, 2025. https://www.ragu.com/our-sauces/ragu-simply/ragu-simply-traditional-sauce

380 LaCroix Pamplemousse Naturally Essenced Sparkling Water. LaCroix Beverages. Accessed April 22, 2025. https://www.lacroixwater.com/flavors/pamplemousse/

381 Coca-Cola® Original. The Coca-Cola Company. Accessed April 22, 2025. https://www.coca-cola.com/us/en/brands/coca-cola/products/original

382 Popkin BM, Armstrong LE, Bray GM, Caballero B, Frei B, Willett WC. A new proposed guidance system for beverage consumption in the United States. *Am J Clin Nutr*. 2006;83(3):529–42. doi: 10.1093/ajcn.83.3.529

383 Morgado M, Ascenso C, Carmo J, Mendes JJ, Manso AC. pH analysis of still and carbonated bottled water: potential influence on dental erosion. *Clin Exp Dent Res*. 2022;8(2):552–60. doi: 10.1002/cre2.535

384 Agro C, Cowley J. Marketplace tested Perrier, LaCroix, Bubly sparkling waters to see which is most acidicic. CBC News. November 14, 2021. Accessed April 17, 2025. https://www.cbc.ca/news/canada/marketplace-carbonated-water-test-1.6245588

385 Mariotti F. Nutritional and health benefits and risks of plant-based substitute foods. *Proc Nutr Soc*. 2025;84(1):110–23. doi: 10.1017/S0029665123004767

386 Whipple T. Is ultra-processed food bad for you? Not always, scientists say. *The Times*. September 28, 2023. Accessed April 17, 2025. https://www.thetimes.com/uk/healthcare/article/is-ultra-processed-food-bad-for-you-not-always-scientists-say-jd05qflg5

387 Levine AS, Ubbink J. Ultra-processed foods: processing versus formulation. *Obes Sci Pract*. 2023;9(4):435–9. doi: 10.1002/osp4.657

388 Gavine A, Shinwell SC, Buchanan P, et al. Support for healthy breastfeeding mothers with healthy term babies. *Cochrane Database Syst Rev*. 2022;10(10):CD001141. doi: 10.1002/14651858.CD001141.pub6

389 Astrup A, Monteiro CA. Does the concept of "ultra-processed foods" help inform dietary guidelines, beyond conventional classification systems? NO. *Am J Clin Nutr*. 2022;116(6):1482–8. doi: 10.1093/ajcn/nqac123

390 Messina M, Sievenpiper JL, Williamson P, Kiel J, Erdman JW Jr. Perspective: soy-based meat and dairy alternatives, despite classification as ultra-processed foods, deliver high-quality nutrition on par with unprocessed or minimally processed animal-based counterparts. *Adv Nutr*. 2022;13(3):726–38. doi: 10.1093/advances/nmac026

391 Consumer perceptions unwrapped: ultra-processed foods. EIT Food. February 1, 2024. Accessed April 17, 2025. https://www.eitfood.eu/reports/ultra-processed-foods

392 Messina M, Sievenpiper JL, Williamson P, Kiel J, Erdman JW Jr. Perspective: soy-based meat and dairy alternatives, despite classification as ultra-processed foods, deliver high-quality nutrition on par with unprocessed or minimally processed animal-based counterparts. *Adv Nutr*. 2022;13(3):726–38. doi: 10.1093/advances/nmac026

393 Wiss DA, LaFata EM. Ultra-processed foods and mental health: where do eating disorders fit into the puzzle? *Nutrients*. 2024;16(12):1955. doi: 10.3390/nu16121955

394 Ulucanlar S, Lauber K, Fabbri A, et al. Corporate political activity: taxonomies and model of corporate influence on public policy. *Int J Health Policy Manag*. 2023;12:7292. doi: 10.34172/ijhpm.2023.7292.

395 Messina MJ, Sievenpiper JL, Williamson P, Kiel J, Erdman JW. Ultra-processed foods: a concept in need of revision to avoid targeting healthful and sustainable plant-based foods. *Public Health Nutr*. 2023;26(7):1390–1. doi: 10.1017/S1368980023000617

396 Lawrence M. The need for particular scrutiny of claims made by researchers associated with ultra-processed food manufacturers. *Br J Nutr*. 2023;130(8):1469–70. doi: 10.1017/S0007114523000429

397 Lawrence M. The need for particular scrutiny of claims made by researchers associated with ultra-processed food manufacturers. *Br J Nutr*. 2023;130(8):1469–70. doi: 10.1017/S0007114523000429

398 Messina MJ, Sievenpiper JL, Williamson P, Kiel J, Erdman JW. Ultra-processed foods: a concept in need of revision to avoid targeting healthful and sustainable plant-based foods. *Public Health Nutr*. 2023;26(7):1390–1. doi: 10.1017/S1368980023000617

399 Messina MJ, Sievenpiper JL, Williamson P, Kiel J, Erdman JW. Ultra-processed foods: a concept in need of revision to avoid targeting healthful and sustainable plant-based foods. *Public Health Nutr*. 2023;26(7):1390–1. doi: 10.1017/S1368980023000617

400 Messina MJ, Sievenpiper JL, Williamson P, Kiel J, Erdman JW. Ultra-processed foods: a concept in need of revision to avoid targeting healthful and sustainable plant-based foods. *Public Health Nutr*. 2023;26(7):1390–1. doi: 10.1017/S1368980023000617

401 Fardet A. Ultra-processing should be understood as a holistic issue, from food matrix, to dietary patterns, food scoring, and food systems. *J Food Sci*. 2024;89(7):4563–73. doi: 10.1111/1750-3841.17139

402 Mozaffarian D, El-Abbadi NH, O'Hearn M, et al. Food Compass is a nutrient profiling system using expanded characteristics for assessing healthfulness of foods. *Nat Food*. 2021;2(10):809–18. doi: 10.1038/s43016-021-00381-y

403 Kellogg's Froot Loops with Fruity Shaped Marshmallows cereal. EatThisMuch.com. Accessed October 3, 2025. https://www.eatthismuch.com/calories/froot-loops-with-fruity-shaped-marshmallows-cereal-2096648

404 Mozaffarian D, El-Abbadi NH, O'Hearn M, et al. Food Compass is a nutrient profiling system using expanded characteristics for assessing healthfulness of foods. *Nat Food*. 2021;2(10):809–18. doi: 10.1038/s43016-021-00381-y

405 Astrup A, Monteiro CA. Does the concept of "ultra-processed foods" help inform dietary guidelines, beyond conventional classification systems? NO. *Am J Clin Nutr*. 2022;116(6):1482–8. doi: 10.1093/ajcn/nqac123

406 Harnack LJ, Reese MM, Johnson AJ. Are plant-based meat alternative products healthier than the animal meats they mimic? *Nutr Today*. 2022;57(4):195–9. doi: 10.1097/NT.0000000000000553

407 Liu AG, Ford NA, Hu FB, Zelman KM, Mozaffarian D, Kris-Etherton PM. A healthy approach to dietary fats: understanding the science and taking action to reduce consumer confusion. *Nutr J*. 2017;16(1):53. doi: 10.1186/s12937-017-0271-4

408 Mozaffarian D, El-Abbadi NH, O'Hearn M, et al. Food Compass is a nutrient profiling system using expanded characteristics for assessing healthfulness of foods. *Nat Food*. 2021;2(10):809–18. doi: 10.1038/s43016-021-00381-y

409 Mozaffarian D, El-Abbadi NH, O'Hearn M, et al. Food Compass is a nutrient profiling system using expanded characteristics for assessing healthfulness of foods. *Nat Food*. 2021;2(10):809–18. doi: 10.1038/s43016-021-00381-y

410 Mozaffarian D, El-Abbadi NH, O'Hearn M, et al. Food Compass is a nutrient profiling system using expanded characteristics for assessing healthfulness of foods. *Nat Food*. 2021;2(10):809–18. doi: 10.1038/s43016-021-00381-y

411 Mozaffarian D, El-Abbadi NH, O'Hearn M, et al. Food Compass is a nutrient profiling system using expanded characteristics for assessing healthfulness of foods. *Nat Food*. 2021;2(10):809–18. doi: 10.1038/s43016-021-00381-y

412 Jones A, Rådholm K, Neal B. Defining 'unhealthy': a systematic analysis of alignment between the Australian Dietary Guidelines and the Health Star Rating System. *Nutrients*. 2018;10(4):501. doi: 10.3390/nu10040501

413 Health Star Rating System. Australian Government. Accessed April 22, 2025. https://www.healthstarrating.gov.au/shoppers

414 Jones A, Rådholm K, Neal B. Defining 'unhealthy': a systematic analysis of alignment between the Australian Dietary Guidelines and the Health Star Rating System. *Nutrients*. 2018;10(4):501. doi: 10.3390/nu10040501

415 Mozaffarian D, El-Abbadi NH, O'Hearn M, et al. Food Compass is a nutrient profiling system using expanded characteristics for assessing healthfulness of foods. *Nat Food*. 2021;2(10):809–18. doi: 10.1038/s43016-021-00381-y

416 Mozaffarian D, El-Abbadi NH, O'Hearn M, et al. Food Compass is a nutrient profiling system using expanded characteristics for assessing healthfulness of foods. *Nat Food*. 2021;2(10):809–18. doi: 10.1038/s43016-021-00381-y

417 Hercberg S, Touvier M, Salas-Salvado J, et al. The Nutri-Score nutrition label: a public health tool based on rigorous scientific evidence aiming to improve the nutritional status of the population. *Int J Vitam Nutr Res*. 2022;92(3-4):147–57. doi: 10.1024/0300-9831/a000722

418 Besancon S, Beran D, Batal M. A study is 21 times more likely to find unfavourable results about the nutrition label Nutri-Score if the authors declare a conflict of interest or the study is funded by the food industry. *BMJ Glob Health*. 2023;8(5). doi: 10.1136/bmjgh-2023-011720

419 Mozaffarian D, El-Abbadi NH, O'Hearn M, et al. Food Compass is a nutrient profiling system using expanded characteristics for assessing healthfulness of foods. *Nat Food*. 2021;2(10):809–18. doi: 10.1038/s43016-021-00381-y

420 Lee JJ, Srebot S, Ahmed M, Mulligan C, Hu G, L'Abbé MR. Nutritional quality and price of plant-based dairy and meat analogs in the Canadian food supply system. *J Food Sci*. 2023;88(8):3594–606. doi: 10.1111/1750-3841.16691

421 Alessandrini R, Brown MK, Pombo-Rodrigues S, Bhageerutty S, He FJ, MacGregor GA. Nutritional quality of plant-based meat products available in the UK: a cross-sectional survey. *Nutrients*. 2021;13(12):4225. doi: 10.3390/nu13124225

422 Zhang L, Langlois E, Williams K, et al. A comparative analysis of nutritional quality, amino acid profile, and nutritional supplementations in plant-based products and their animal-based counterparts in the UK. *Food Chem*. 2024;448:139059. doi: 10.1016/j.foodchem.2024.139059

423 Cutroneo S, Angelino D, Tedeschi T, Pellegrini N, Martini D; SINU Young Working Group. nutritional quality of meat analogues: results from the Food Labelling of Italian Products (FLIP) Project. *Front Nutr*. 2022;9:852831. doi: 10.3389/fnut.2022.852831

424 Kalocsay K, King T, Lichtenstein T, Weber J. *Plant-Based Meat: A Healthier Choice?* Food Frontier; 2020. https://www.foodfrontier.org/resource/plant-based-meat-a-healthier-choice/

425 Locatelli NT, Chen GFN, Batista MF, et al. Nutrition classification schemes for plant-based meat analogues: drivers to assess nutritional quality and identity profile. *Curr Res Food Sci*. 2024;9:100796. doi: 10.1016/j.crfs.2024.100796

426 de las Heras-Delgado S, Shyam S, Cunillera È, Dragusan N, Salas-Salvadó J, Babio N. Are plant-based alternatives healthier? A two-dimensional evaluation from nutritional and processing standpoints. *Food Res Int*. 2023;169:112857. doi: 10.1016/j.foodres.2023.112857

427 Petersen T, Hartmann M, Hirsch S. Which meat (substitute) to buy? Is front of package information reliable to identify the healthier and more natural choice? *Food Qual Prefer*. 2021;94:104298. doi: 10.1016/j.foodqual.2021.104298

428 Lindberg L, McCann RR, Smyth B, Woodside JV, Nugent AP. The environmental impact, ingredient composition, nutritional and health impact of meat alternatives: a systematic review. *Trends Food Sci Technol*. 2024;149:104483. doi: 10.1016/j.tifs.2024.104483

429 Springmann M. A multicriteria analysis of meat and milk alternatives from nutritional, health, environmental, and cost perspectives. *Proc Natl Acad Sci USA*. 2024;121(50):e2319010121. doi: 10.1073/pnas.2319010121

430 Lindberg L, McCann RR, Smyth B, Woodside JV, Nugent AP. The environmental impact, ingredient composition, nutritional and health impact of meat alternatives: a systematic review. *Trends Food Sci Technol*. 2024;149:104483. doi: 10.1016/j.tifs.2024.104483

431 Monteiro CA. Letters to the editor. *Public Health Nutr*. 2009;12(10):1968–9. doi: 10.1017/S1368980009991212

432 Lindberg L, McCann RR, Smyth B, Woodside JV, Nugent AP. The environmental impact, ingredient composition, nutritional and health impact of meat alternatives: a systematic review. *Trends Food Sci Technol*. 2024;149:104483. doi: 10.1016/j.tifs.2024.104483

433 Astrup A, Monteiro CA. Does the concept of "ultra-processed foods" help inform dietary guidelines, beyond conventional classification systems? NO. *Am J Clin Nutr*. 2022;116(6):1482–8. doi: 10.1093/ajcn/nqac123

434 NECTAR Taste of the Industry 2024. Food System Innovations. June 2024. Accessed April 23, 2025. https://www.nectar.org/sensory-research/2024-taste-of-the-industry

435 McClements IF, McClements DJ. Designing healthier plant-based foods: fortification, digestion, and bioavailability. *Food Res Int*. 2023;169:112853. doi: 10.1016/j.foodres.2023.112853

436 NECTAR Taste of the Industry 2024. Food System Innovations. June 2024. Accessed April 23, 2025. https://www.nectar.org/sensory-research/2024-taste-of-the-industry

437 Astrup A, Monteiro CA. Does the concept of "ultra-processed foods" help inform dietary guidelines, beyond conventional classification systems? NO. *Am J Clin Nutr*. 2022;116(6):1482–8. doi: 10.1093/ajcn/nqac123

438 Touvier M, da Costa Louzada ML, Mozaffarian D, Baker P, Juul F, Srour B. Ultra-processed foods and cardiometabolic health: public health policies to reduce consumption cannot wait. *BMJ*. 2023;383:e075294. doi: 10.1136/bmj-2023-075294

439 Zinöcker MK, Lindseth IA. The Western diet-microbiome-host interaction and its role in metabolic disease. *Nutrients*. 2018;10(3):365. doi: 10.3390/nu10030365

440 Grundy MM, Carrière F, Mackie AR, Gray DA, Butterworth PJ, Ellis PR. The role of plant cell wall encapsulation and porosity in regulating lipolysis during the digestion of almond seeds. *Food Funct*. 2016;7(1):69–78. doi: 10.1039/c5fo00758e

441 Zinöcker MK, Lindseth IA. The Western diet-microbiome-host interaction and its role in metabolic disease. *Nutrients*. 2018;10(3):365. doi: 10.3390/nu10030365

442 Astrup A, Monteiro CA. Does the concept of "ultra-processed foods" help inform dietary guidelines, beyond conventional classification systems? NO. *Am J Clin Nutr*. 2022;116(6):1482–8. doi: 10.1093/ajcn/nqac123

443 Monjotin N, Amiot MJ, Fleurentin J, Morel JM, Raynal S. Clinical evidence of the benefits of phytonutrients in human healthcare. *Nutrients*. 2022;14(9):1712. doi: 10.3390/nu14091712

444 Scheier L. Salicylic acid: one more reason to eat your fruits and vegetables. *J Am Diet Assoc*. 2001;101(12):1406–8. doi: 10.1016/S0002-8223(01)00337-6

445 van Vliet S, Bain JR, Muehlbauer MJ, et al. A metabolomics comparison of plant-based meat and grass-fed meat indicates large nutritional differences despite comparable Nutrition Facts panels. *Sci Rep*. 2021;11(1):13828. doi: 10.1038/s41598-021-93100-3

446 Astrup A, Monteiro CA. Does the concept of "ultra-processed foods" help inform dietary guidelines, beyond conventional classification systems? NO. *Am J Clin Nutr*. 2022;116(6):1482–8. doi: 10.1093/ajcn/nqac123

447 van Vliet S, Provenza FD, Kronberg SL. Health-promoting phytonutrients are higher in grass-fed meat and milk. *Front Sustain Food Syst*. 2021;4:555426. doi: 10.3389/fsufs.2020.555426

448 Descalzo AM, Insani EM, Biolatto A, et al. Influence of pasture or grain-based diets supplemented with vitamin E on antioxidant/oxidative balance of Argentine beef. *Meat Sci.* 2005;70(1):35–44. doi: 10.1016/j.meatsci.2004.11.018

449 Descalzo AM, Rossetti L, Grigioni G, et al. Antioxidant status and odour profile in fresh beef from pasture or grain-fed cattle. *Meat Sci.* 2007;75(2):299–307. doi: 10.1016/j.meatsci.2006.07.015

450 Agricultural Research Service, United States Department of Agriculture. Oranges, raw, navels. FoodData Central. December 2019. Accessed September 19, 2025. https://fdc.nal.usda.gov/food-details/746771/nutrients

451 Descalzo AM, Rossetti L, Grigioni G, et al. Antioxidant status and odour profile in fresh beef from pasture or grain-fed cattle. *Meat Sci.* 2007;75(2):299–307. doi: 10.1016/j.meatsci.2006.07.015

452 Gatellier P, Mercier Y, Renerre M. Effect of diet finishing mode (pasture or mixed diet) on antioxidant status of Charolais bovine meat. *Meat Sci.* 2004;67(3):385–94. doi: 10.1016/j.meatsci.2003.11.009

453 Carlsen MH, Halvorsen BL, Holte K, et al. The total antioxidant content of more than 3100 foods, beverages, spices, herbs and supplements used worldwide. *Nutr J.* 2010;9:3. doi: 10.1186/1475-2891-9-3

454 Carlsen MH, Halvorsen BL, Holte K, et al. The total antioxidant content of more than 3100 foods, beverages, spices, herbs and supplements used worldwide. *Nutr J.* 2010;9:3. doi: 10.1186/1475-2891-9-3

455 Green AS. mTOR, glycotoxins and the parallel universe. *Aging (Albany NY).* 2018;10(12):3654–6. doi: 10.18632/aging.101720

456 Rungratanawanich W, Qu Y, Wang X, Essa MM, Song BJ. Advanced glycation end products (AGEs) and other adducts in aging-related diseases and alcohol-mediated tissue injury. *Exp Mol Med.* 2021;53(2):168–88. doi: 10.1038/s12276-021-00561-7

457 Uribarri J, Woodruff S, Goodman S, et al. Advanced glycation end products in foods and a practical guide to their reduction in the diet. *J Am Diet Assoc.* 2010;110(6):911–6.e12. doi: 10.1016/j.jada.2010.03.018

458 Ishaq A, Irfan S, Sameen A, Khalid N. Plant-based meat analogs: a review with reference to formulation and gastrointestinal fate. *Curr Res Food Sci.* 2022;5:973–83. doi: 10.1016/j.crfs.2022.06.001

459 Scheijen JLJM, Clevers E, Engelen L, Dagnelie PC, Brouns F, Stehouwer CDA, Schalkwijk CG. Analysis of advanced glycation endproducts in selected food items by ultra-performance liquid chromatography tandem mass spectrometry: presentation of a dietary AGE database. *Food Chem.* 2016;190:1145–50. doi: 10.1016/j.foodchem.2015.06.049

460 Hull GLJ, Woodside JV, Ames JM, Cuskelly GJ. Nε-(carboxymethyl)lysine content of foods commonly consumed in a western style diet. *Food Chem.* 2012;131(1):170–4. doi: 10.1016/j.foodchem.2011.08.055

461 Silva Barbosa Correia B, Drud-Heydary Nielsen S, Jorkowski J, Arildsen Jakobsen LM, Zacherl C, Bertram HC. Maillard reaction products and metabolite profile of plant-based meat burgers compared with traditional meat burgers and cooking-induced alterations. *Food Chem.* 2024;445:138705. doi: 10.1016/j.foodchem.2024.138705

462 Deng P, Chen Y, Xie S, et al. Accumulation of heterocyclic amines and advanced glycation end products in various processing stages of plant-based burgers by UHPLC-MS/MS. *J Agric Food Chem*. 2022;70(46):14771–83. doi: 10.1021/acs.jafc.2c06393

463 Li H, Yang H, Li P, et al. Maillard reaction products with furan ring, like furosine, cause kidney injury through triggering ferroptosis pathway. *Food Chem*. 2020;319:126368. doi: 10.1016/j.foodchem.2020.126368

464 Silva Barbosa Correia B, Drud-Heydary Nielsen S, Jorkowski J, Arildsen Jakobsen LM, Zacherl C, Bertram HC. Maillard reaction products and metabolite profile of plant-based meat burgers compared with traditional meat burgers and cooking-induced alterations. *Food Chem*. 2024;445:138705. doi: 10.1016/j.foodchem.2024.138705

465 Laguzzi F, Filippini T, Virgolino A. Editorial: dietary acrylamide in human health. *Front Nutr*. 2024;11:1446690. doi: 10.3389/fnut.2024.1446690

466 Hogervorst JGF, Schouten LJ. Dietary acrylamide and human cancer; even after 20 years of research an open question. *Am J Clin Nutr*. 2022;116(4):846–7. doi: 10.1093/ajcn/nqac192

467 Pospiech J, Hoelzle E, Schoepf A, Melzer T, Granvogl M, Frank J. Acrylamide increases and furanoic compounds decrease in plant-based meat alternatives during pan-frying. *Food Chem*. 2024;439:138063. doi: 10.1016/j.foodchem.2023.138063

468 Fu S, Ma Y, Wang Y, et al. Contents and correlations of $N\varepsilon$-(carboxymethyl)lysine, $N\varepsilon$-(carboxyethyl)lysine, acrylamide and nutrients in plant-based meat analogs. *Foods*. 2023;12(10):1967. doi: 10.3390/foods12101967

469 Pospiech J, Hoelzle E, Schoepf A, Melzer T, Granvogl M, Frank J. Acrylamide increases and furanoic compounds decrease in plant-based meat alternatives during pan-frying. *Food Chem*. 2024;439:138063. doi: 10.1016/j.foodchem.2023.138063

470 Başaran B, Çuvalcı B, Kaban G. Dietary acrylamide exposure and cancer risk: a systematic approach to human epidemiological studies. *Foods*. 2023;12(2):346. doi: 10.3390/foods12020346

471 Nica-Badea D. Relevance of dietary exposure to acrylamide formed in heat-processed agri-food products. *Cent Eur J Public Health*. 2022;30(3):179–84. doi: 10.21101/cejph.a6779

472 Guth S, Baum M, Cartus AT, et al. Evaluation of the genotoxic potential of acrylamide: arguments for the derivation of a tolerable daily intake (TDI value). *Food Chem Toxicol*. 2023;173:113632. doi: 10.1016/j.fct.2023.113632

473 Pospiech J, Hoelzle E, Schoepf A, Melzer T, Granvogl M, Frank J. Acrylamide increases and furanoic compounds decrease in plant-based meat alternatives during pan-frying. *Food Chem*. 2024;439:138063. doi: 10.1016/j.foodchem.2023.138063

474 Filippini T, Halldorsson TI, Capitão C, et al. Dietary acrylamide exposure and risk of site-specific cancer: a systematic review and dose-response meta-analysis of epidemiological studies. *Front Nutr*. 2022;9:875607. doi: 10.3389/fnut.2022.875607

475 Pospiech J, Hoelzle E, Schoepf A, Melzer T, Granvogl M, Frank J. Acrylamide increases and furanoic compounds decrease in plant-based meat alternatives during pan-frying. *Food Chem*. 2024;439:138063. doi: 10.1016/j.foodchem.2023.138063

476 Sasso A, Latella G. Role of heme iron in the association between red meat consumption and colorectal cancer. *Nutr Cancer*. 2018;70(8):1173–83. doi: 10.1080/01635581.2018.1521441

477 Barzegar F, Kamankesh M, Mohammadi A. Heterocyclic aromatic amines in cooked food: a review on formation, health risk-toxicology and their analytical techniques. *Food Chem*. 2019;280:240–54. doi: 10.1016/j.foodchem.2018.12.058

478 Trujillo-Mayol I, Madalena C Sobral M, et al. Incorporation of avocado peel extract to reduce cooking-induced hazards in beef and soy burgers: a clean label ingredient. *Food Res Int*. 2021;147:110434. doi: 10.1016/j.foodres.2021.110434

479 Thiébaud HP, Knize MG, Kuzmicky PA, Hsieh DP, Felton JS. Airborne mutagens produced by frying beef, pork and a soy-based food. *Food Chem Toxicol*. 1995;33(10):821–8. doi: 10.1016/0278-6915(95)00057-9

480 Trujillo-Mayol I, Madalena C Sobral M, et al. Incorporation of avocado peel extract to reduce cooking-induced hazards in beef and soy burgers: a clean label ingredient. *Food Res Int*. 2021;147:110434. doi: 10.1016/j.foodres.2021.110434

481 Deng P, Chen Y, Xie S, et al. Accumulation of heterocyclic amines and advanced glycation end products in various processing stages of plant-based burgers by UHPLC-MS/MS. *J Agric Food Chem*. 2022;70(46):14771–83. doi: 10.1021/acs.jafc.2c06393

482 Xi J, Chen Y. Analysis of the relationship between heterocyclic amines and the oxidation and thermal decomposition of protein using the dry heated soy protein isolate system. *LWT*. 2021;148:111738. doi: 10.1016/j.lwt.2021.111738

483 Bulanda S, Janoszka B. Consumption of thermally processed meat containing carcinogenic compounds (polycyclic aromatic hydrocarbons and heterocyclic aromatic amines) versus a risk of some cancers in humans and the possibility of reducing their formation by natural food additives—a literature review. *Int J Environ Res Public Health*. 2022;19(8):4781. doi: 10.3390/ijerph19084781

484 IARC Working Group on the Evaluation of Carcinogenic Risks to Humans. *Red Meat and Processed Meat*. International Agency for Research on Cancer; 2018. PMID: 29949327.

485 Zastrow L, Speer K, Schwind KH, Jira W. A sensitive GC-HRMS method for the simultaneous determination of parent and oxygenated polycyclic aromatic hydrocarbons in barbecued meat and meat substitutes. *Food Chem*. 2021;365:130625. doi: 10.1016/j.foodchem.2021.130625

486 Sasso A, Latella G. Role of heme iron in the association between red meat consumption and colorectal cancer. *Nutr Cancer*. 2018;70(8):1173–83. doi: 10.1080/01635581.2018.1521441

487 Sasso A, Latella G. Role of heme iron in the association between red meat consumption and colorectal cancer. *Nutr Cancer*. 2018;70(8):1173–83. doi: 10.1080/01635581.2018.1521441

488 IARC Working Group on the Evaluation of Carcinogenic Risks to Humans. *Red Meat and Processed Meat*. International Agency for Research on Cancer; 2018. PMID: 29949327.

489 IARC Working Group on the Evaluation of Carcinogenic Risks to Humans. *Red Meat and Processed Meat*. International Agency for Research on Cancer; 2018. PMID: 29949327.

490 Chan SE, Smith CA. A food product as a potential serious cause of liver injury. *Clin Toxicol*. 2023;61(8):616–9. doi: 10.1080/15563650.2023.2256469

491 Sebranek JG, Jackson-Davis AL, Myers KL, Lavieri NA. Beyond celery and starter culture: advances in natural/organic curing processes in the United States. *Meat Sci.* 2012;92(3):267–73. doi: 10.1016/j.meatsci.2012.03.002

492 Sofos JN, Busta FF, Allen CE. Botulism control by nitrite and sorbate in cured meats: a review. *J Food Prot.* 1979;42(9):739–70. doi: 10.4315/0362-028X-42.9.739

493 Astrup A, Monteiro CA. Does the concept of "ultra-processed foods" help inform dietary guidelines, beyond conventional classification systems? NO. *Am J Clin Nutr.* 2022;116(6):1482–8. doi: 10.1093/ajcn/nqac123

494 IARC Working Group on the Evaluation of Carcinogenic Risks to Humans. *Red Meat and Processed Meat.* International Agency for Research on Cancer; 2018. PMID: 29949327.

495 Fraser RZ, Shitut M, Agrawal P, Mendes O, Klapholz S. Safety evaluation of soy leghemoglobin protein preparation derived from *Pichia pastoris*, intended for use as a flavor catalyst in plant-based meat. *Int J Toxicol.* 2018;37(3):241–62. doi: 10.1177/1091581818766318

496 Flink T. What's vegan at Burger King? The complete menu guide. *VegNews.* September 8, 2025. Accessed October 8, 2025. https://vegnews.com/guides/vegan-guide-burger-king

497 Turner ND, Lloyd SK. Association between red meat consumption and colon cancer: a systematic review of experimental results. *Exp Biol Med.* 2017;242(8):813–39. doi: 10.1177/1535370217693117

498 World Cancer Research Fund/American Institute for Cancer Research. *Diet, Nutrition, Physical Activity and Cancer: A Global Perspective.* World Cancer Research Fund International; 2017. Revised 2018. Accessed May 15, 2025. https://www.wcrf.org/wp-content/uploads/2024/10/Colorectal-cancer-report.pdf

499 Astrup A, Monteiro CA. Does the concept of "ultra-processed foods" help inform dietary guidelines, beyond conventional classification systems? NO. *Am J Clin Nutr.* 2022;116(6):1482–8. doi: 10.1093/ajcn/nqac123

500 Petersen T, Hartmann M, Hirsch S. Which meat (substitute) to buy? Is front of package information reliable to identify the healthier and more natural choice? *Food Qual.* 2021;94:104298. doi: 10.1016/j.foodqual.2021.104298

501 Lindberg L, McCann RR, Smyth B, Woodside JV, Nugent AP. The environmental impact, ingredient composition, nutritional and health impact of meat alternatives: a systematic review. *Trends Food Sci Technol.* 2024;149:104483. doi: 10.1016/j.tifs.2024.104483

502 Codex Alimentarius Commission. Methyl cellulose. Codex General Standard for Food Additives (GSFA) Online Database. 2024. Accessed April 23, 2025. https://www.fao.org/gsfaonline/additives/details.html?id=83

503 Ewart MH, Chapman RA. Identification of stabilizing agents. *Anal Chem.* 1952;24(9):1460–4. http://lib3.dss.go.th/fulltext/scan_ebook/ana_1952_v24_no9.pdf

504 Bampidis V, Azimonti G, Bastos ML,. Safety and efficacy of methyl cellulose for all animal species. *EFSA J.* 2020;18(7):e06212. doi: 10.2903/j.efsa.2020.6212

505 Younes M, Aggett P, Aguilar F, et al. Re-evaluation of celluloses E 460(i), E 460(ii), E 461, E 462, E 463, E 464, E 465, E 466, E 468 and E 469 as food additives. *EFSA J.* 2018;16(1):e05047. doi: 10.2903/j.efsa.2018.5047

506 Whelan K, Bancil AS, Lindsay JO, Chassaing B. Ultra-processed foods and food additives in gut health and disease. *Nat Rev Gastroenterol Hepatol*. 2024;21(6):406–27. doi: 10.1038/s41575-024-00893-5

507 Swidsinski A, Ung V, Sydora BC, at al. Bacterial overgrowth and inflammation of small intestine after carboxymethylcellulose ingestion in genetically susceptible mice. *Inflamm Bowel Dis*. 2009;15(3):359–64. doi: 10.1002/ibd.20763

508 Rousta E, Oka A, Liu B, et al. The emulsifier carboxymethylcellulose induces more aggressive colitis in humanized mice with inflammatory bowel disease microbiota than polysorbate-80. *Nutrients*. 2021;13(10):3565. doi: 10.3390/nu13103565

509 Delaroque C, Chassaing B. Dietary emulsifier consumption accelerates type 1 diabetes development in NOD mice. *NPJ Biofilms Microbiomes*. 2024;10(1):1. doi: 10.1038/s41522-023-00475-4

510 Viennois E, Chassaing B. Consumption of select dietary emulsifiers exacerbates the development of spontaneous intestinal adenoma. *Int J Mol Sci*. 2021;22(5):2602. doi: 10.3390/ijms22052602

511 Viennois E, Merlin D, Gewirtz AT, Chassaing B. Dietary emulsifier-induced low-grade inflammation promotes colon carcinogenesis. *Cancer Res*. 2017;77(1):27–40. doi: 10.1158/0008-5472.CAN-16-1359

512 Harusato A, Chassaing B, Dauriat CJG, Ushiroda C, Seo W, Itoh Y. Dietary emulsifiers exacerbate food allergy and colonic type 2 immune response through microbiota modulation. *Nutrients*. 2022;14(23):4983. doi: 10.3390/nu14234983

513 Panyod S, Wu WK, Chang CT, et al. Common dietary emulsifiers promote metabolic disorders and intestinal microbiota dysbiosis in mice. *Commun Biol*. 2024;7(1):749. doi: 10.1038/s42003-024-06224-3

514 Holder MK, Peters NV, Whylings J, Fields CT, Gewirtz AT, Chassaing B, de Vries GJ. Dietary emulsifiers consumption alters anxiety-like and social-related behaviors in mice in a sex-dependent manner. *Sci Rep*. 2019;9(1):172. doi: 10.1038/s41598-018-36890-3

515 Milà-Guasch M, Ramírez S, Llana SR, et al. Maternal emulsifier consumption programs offspring metabolic and neuropsychological health in mice. *PLoS Biol*. 2023;21(8):e3002171. doi: 10.1371/journal.pbio.3002171

516 Lock JY, Carlson TL, Wang CM, Chen A, Carrier RL. Acute exposure to commonly ingested emulsifiers alters intestinal mucus structure and transport properties. *Sci Rep*. 2018;8(1):10008. doi: 10.1038/s41598-018-27957-2

517 Viennois E, Chassaing B. First victim, later aggressor: how the intestinal microbiota drives the pro-inflammatory effects of dietary emulsifiers? *Gut Microbes*. 2018;9(3):1–4. doi: 10.1080/19490976.2017.1421885

518 Harusato A, Chassaing B, Dauriat CJG, Ushiroda C, Seo W, Itoh Y. Dietary emulsifiers exacerbate food allergy and colonic type 2 immune response through microbiota modulation. *Nutrients*. 2022;14(23):4983. doi: 10.3390/nu14234983

519 Whelan K, Bancil AS, Lindsay JO, Chassaing B. Ultra-processed foods and food additives in gut health and disease. *Nat Rev Gastroenterol Hepatol*. 2024;21(6):406–27. doi: 10.1038/s41575-024-00893-5

520 Levine A, Rhodes JM, Lindsay JO, et al. Dietary guidance from the International Organization for the Study of Inflammatory Bowel Diseases. *Clin Gastroenterol Hepatol*. 2020;18(6):1381–92. doi: 10.1016/j.cgh.2020.01.046

521 Chassaing B, Compher C, Bonhomme B, et al. Randomized controlled-feeding study of dietary emulsifier carboxymethylcellulose reveals detrimental impacts on the gut microbiota and metabolome. *Gastroenterology*. 2022;162(3):743–56. doi: 10.1053/j. gastro.2021.11.006

522 Chassaing B, Van de Wiele T, De Bodt J, Marzorati M, Gewirtz AT. Dietary emulsifiers directly alter human microbiota composition and gene expression ex vivo potentiating intestinal inflammation. *Gut*. 2017;66(8):1414–27. doi: 10.1136/gutjnl-2016-313099

523 Bhattacharyya S, Shumard T, Xie H, et al. A randomized trial of the effects of the no-carrageenan diet on ulcerative colitis disease activity. *Nutr Healthy Aging*. 2017;4(2):181–92. doi: 10.3233/NHA-170023

524 Fitzpatrick JA, Gibson PR, Taylor KM, Halmos EP. The effect of dietary emulsifiers and thickeners on intestinal barrier function and its response to acute stress in healthy adult humans: a randomised controlled feeding study. *Aliment Pharmacol Ther*. 2024;60(7):863–75. doi: 10.1111/apt.18172

525 Chassaing B, Compher C, Bonhomme B, et al. Randomized controlled-feeding study of dietary emulsifier carboxymethylcellulose reveals detrimental impacts on the gut microbiota and metabolome. *Gastroenterology*. 2022;162(3):743–56. doi: 10.1053/j. gastro.2021.11.006

526 Hamilton JW, Wagner J, Burdick BB, Bass P. Clinical evaluation of methylcellulose as a bulk laxative. *Dig Dis Sci*. 1988;33(8):993–8. doi: 10.1007/BF01535996

527 Swartz ML. Citrucel (methylcellulose/bulk-forming laxative). *Gastroenterol Nurs*. 1989;12(1):50–2. doi: 10.1097/00001610-198907000-00013

528 Citrucel Orange Flavor Methylcellulose Fiber Therapy. Citrucel. Accessed April 23, 2025. https://www.citrucel.com/products/orange-mix-powder/

529 Citrucel: methylcellulose fiber therapy for regularity with smartfiber. Medshopexpress. Accessed October 8, 2025. https://www.medshopexpress.com/citrucel-methylcellulose-fiber-therapy-for-regularity-with-smartfiber-240-caplets

530 Whelan K, Bancil AS, Lindsay JO, Chassaing B. Ultra-processed foods and food additives in gut health and disease. *Nat Rev Gastroenterol Hepatol*. 2024;21(6):406–27. doi: 10.1038/s41575-024-00893-5

531 Salame C, Javaux G, Sellem L, et al. Food additive emulsifiers and the risk of type 2 diabetes: analysis of data from the NutriNet-Santé prospective cohort study. *Lancet Diabetes Endocrinol*. 2024;12(5):339–49. doi: 10.1016/S2213-8587(24)00086-X

532 Sellem L, Srour B, Javaux G, Chazelas E, Chassaing B, Viennois E, Debras C, Salamé C, Druesne-Pecollo N, Esseddik Y, de Edelenyi FS, Agaësse C, De Sa A, Lutchia R, Louveau E, Huybrechts I, Pierre F, Coumoul X, Fezeu LK, Julia C, Kesse-Guyot E, Allès B, Galan P, Hercberg S, Deschasaux-Tanguy M, Touvier M. Food additive emulsifiers and risk of cardiovascular disease in the NutriNet-Santé cohort: prospective cohort study. *BMJ*. 2023;382:e076058. doi: 10.1136/bmj-2023-076058

533 Miclotte L, De Paepe K, Rymenans L, Callewaert C, Raes J, Rajkovic A, Van Camp J, Van de Wiele T. Dietary emulsifiers alter composition and activity of the human gut microbiota *in vitro*, irrespective of chemical or natural emulsifier origin. *Front Microbiol*. 2020;11:577474. doi: 10.3389/fmicb.2020.577474

534 Naimi S, Viennois E, Gewirtz AT, Chassaing B. Direct impact of commonly used dietary emulsifiers on human gut microbiota. *Microbiome.* 2021;9(1):66. doi: 10.1186/s40168-020-00996-6

535 Navratilova HF, Whetton AD, Geifman N. Plant-based meat alternatives intake and its association with health status among vegetarians of the UK Biobank volunteer population. *Food Frontiers.* 2025;6(1):590–8. doi: 10.1002/fft2.532

536 Beach C. FDA determines that tara flour is not safe; 500 were sickened by the ingredient. *Food Safety News.* May 16, 2024. Accessed April 24, 2025. https://www.foodsafetynews.com/2024/05/fda-determines-that-tara-flour-is-not-safe-500-were-sickened-by-the-ingredient/

537 Choi G, Ahmad J, Navarro V, et al. Characterisation of an outbreak of acute liver injury after ingestion of plant-based food supplement. *Aliment Pharmacol Ther.* 2024;60(4):479–83. doi: 10.1111/apt.18116

538 FDA Coordinated Outbreak Response & Evaluation Network. *Incident Summary Report: Adverse Illness Event Series/Lentil and Leek Crumbles/June 2022 (CARA #1076).* October 18, 2022. Accessed April 24, 2025. https://foodfix.co/wp-content/uploads/Daily-Harvest-Outbreak-FDA-Records.pdf

539 Chittiboyina AG, Ali Z, Avula B, et al. Is baikiain in tara flour a causative agent for the adverse events associated with the recalled frozen French Lentil & Leek Crumbles food product?—a working hypothesis. *Chem Res Toxicol.* 2023;36(6):818–21. doi: 10.1021/acs.chemrestox.3c00100

540 U.S. Food & Drug Administration, Center for Food Safety and Applied Nutrition. Regulatory status and review of available information pertaining to tara protein/flour derived from the seed germ of the plant, Caesalpinia spinosa: lack of general recognition of safety for its use in foods. U.S. Food & Drug Administration. April 10, 2024. Accessed October 8, 2025. https://www.fda.gov/food/hfp-constituent-updates/fda-update-post-market-assessment-tara-flour

541 Fierro O, Siano F, Bianco M, Vasca E, Picariello G. Comprehensive molecular level characterization of protein- and polyphenol-rich tara (*Caesalpinia spinosa*) seed germ flour suggests novel hypothesis about possible accidental hazards. *Food Res Int.* 2024;181:114119. doi: 10.1016/J.foodres.2024.114119

542 A discussion of tara and GRAS status. Food Safety News. August 5, 2022. Accessed April 24, 2025. https://www.foodsafetynews.com/2022/08/a-discussion-of-tara-and-gras-status/

543 FDA Coordinated Outbreak Response & Evaluation Network. *Incident Summary Report: Adverse Illness Event Series/Lentil and Leek Crumbles/June 2022 (CARA #1076).* October 18, 2022. Accessed April 24, 2025. https://foodfix.co/wp-content/uploads/Daily-Harvest-Outbreak-FDA-Records.pdf

544 Chan SE, Smith CA. A food product as a potential serious cause of liver injury. *Clin Toxicol.* 2023;61(8):616–9. doi: 10.1080/15563650.2023.2256469

545 Choi G, Ahmad J, Navarro V, et al. Characterisation of an outbreak of acute liver injury after ingestion of plant-based food supplement. *Aliment Pharmacol Ther.* 2024;60(4):479–83. doi: 10.1111/apt.18116

546 Gaumnitz J, DuBroff J, Aguilar M. S3752—novel case of tara flour-induced liver injury. *Am J Gastroenterol.* 2023;118(10S):S2420-S2420. doi: 10.14309/01.ajg.0000964648.61550.ec

547 Cohen PA, Broad Leib EM. Ingesting risk—the FDA and new food ingredients. *N Engl J Med*. 2024;391(10):875–7. doi: 10.1056/NEJMp2403165

548 Chittiboyina AG, Ali Z, Avula B, et al. Is baikiain in tara flour a causative agent for the adverse events associated with the recalled frozen French Lentil & Leek Crumbles food product?—a working hypothesis. *Chem Res Toxicol*. 2023;36(6):818–21. doi: 10.1021/acs.chemrestox.3c00100

549 Fierro O, Siano F, Bianco M, Vasca E, Picariello G. Comprehensive molecular level characterization of protein- and polyphenol-rich tara (*Caesalpinia spinosa*) seed germ flour suggests novel hypothesis about possible accidental hazards. *Food Res Int*. 2024;181:114119. doi: 10.1016/j.foodres.2024.114119

550 U.S. Food and Drug Administration. FDA update on the post-market assessment of tara flour. May 15, 2024. Accessed April 24, 2025. https://www.fda.gov/food/hfp-constituent-updates/fda-update-post-market-assessment-tara-flour

551 Canadian Food Inspection Agency. Notice to industry: tara protein powder (tara flour) not assessed for safety by Health Canada. September 28, 2023. Accessed April 24, 2025. https://inspection.canada.ca/en/importing-food-plants-animals/food-imports/food-import-notices-industry/2023-09-28

552 U.S. Food and Drug Administration. FDA update on the post-market assessment of tara flour. May 15, 2024. Accessed April 24, 2025. https://www.fda.gov/food/hfp-constituent-updates/fda-update-post-market-assessment-tara-flour

553 Cohen PA, Broad Leib EM. Ingesting risk—the FDA and new food ingredients. *N Engl J Med*. 2024;391(10):875–7. doi: 10.1056/NEJMp2403165

554 Warren B, Mandeville K. Trans fat elimination (English). *Health, Nutrition and Population (HNP) Knowledge Brief*. World Bank Group; 2022. Accessed April 24, 2025. http://documents.worldbank.org/curated/en/099539110122222880

555 Cohen PA, Broad Leib EM. Ingesting risk—the FDA and new food ingredients. *N Engl J Med*. 2024;391(10):875–7. doi: 10.1056/NEJMp2403165

556 Choi G, Ahmad J, Navarro V, et al. Characterisation of an outbreak of acute liver injury after ingestion of plant-based food supplement. *Aliment Pharmacol Ther*. 2024;60(4):479–83. doi: 10.1111/apt.18116

557 GBD 2017 Diet Collaborators. Health effects of dietary risks in 195 countries, 1990-2017: a systematic analysis for the Global Burden of Disease Study 2017. *Lancet*. 2019;393(10184):1958–72. doi: 10.1016/S0140-6736(19)30041-8

558 Romão B, Botelho RBA, Nakano EY, et al. Are vegan alternatives to meat products healthy? A study on nutrients and main ingredients of products commercialized in Brazil. *Front Public Health*. 2022;10:900598. doi: 10.3389/fpubh.2022.900598

559 Ruusunen M, Puolanne E. Reducing sodium intake from meat products. *Meat Sci*. 2005;70(3):531–41. doi: 10.1016/j.meatsci.2004.07.016

560 National Cancer Institute. *Identification of Top Food Sources of Various Dietary Components*. Epidemiology and Genomics Research Program; 2010. Updated November 30, 2019. Accessed April 16, 2025. https://epi.grants.cancer.gov/diet/foodsources

561 Conis E. The hidden salt in chicken. *Los Angeles Times*. June 22, 2009. Accessed April 24, 2025. https://www.latimes.com/archives/la-xpm-2009-jun-22-he-nutrition22-story.html

562 Lee JJ, Srebot S, Ahmed M, Mulligan C, Hu G, L'Abbé MR. Nutritional quality and price of plant-based dairy and meat analogs in the Canadian food supply system. *J Food Sci*. 2023;88(8):3594–606. doi: 10.1111/1750-3841.16691

563 Coffey AA, Lillywhite R, Oyebode O. Meat versus meat alternatives: which is better for the environment and health? A nutritional and environmental analysis of animal-based products compared with their plant-based alternatives. *J Hum Nutr Diet*. 2023;36(6):2147–56. doi: 10.1111/jhn.13219

564 Romão B, Botelho RBA, Nakano EY, et al. Are vegan alternatives to meat products healthy? A study on nutrients and main ingredients of products commercialized in Brazil. *Front Public Health*. 2022;10:900598. doi: 10.3389/fpubh.2022.900598

565 Melville H, Shahid M, Gaines A, et al. The nutritional profile of plant-based meat analogues available for sale in Australia. *Nutr Diet*. 2023;80(2):211–22. doi: 10.1111/1747-0080.12793

566 Curtain F, Grafenauer S. Plant-based meat substitutes in the flexitarian age: an audit of products on supermarket shelves. *Nutrients*. 2019;11(11):2603. doi: 10.3390/nu11112603

567 Bryngelsson S, Moshtaghian H, Bianchi M, Hallström E. Nutritional assessment of plant-based meat analogues on the Swedish market. *Int J Food Sci Nutr*. 2022;73(7):889–901. doi: 10.1080/09637486.2022.2078286

568 Petersen T, Hartmann M, Hirsch S. Which meat (substitute) to buy? Is front of package information reliable to identify the healthier and more natural choice? *Food Qual*. 2021;94:104298. doi: 10.1016/j.foodqual.2021.104298

569 Salomé M, Huneau JF, Le Baron C, Kesse-Guyot E, Fouillet H, Mariotti F. Substituting meat or dairy products with plant-based substitutes has small and heterogeneous effects on diet quality and nutrient security: a simulation study in French adults (INCA3). *J Nutr*. 2021;151(8):2435–45. doi: 10.1093/jn/nxab146

570 Petersen T, Hirsch S. Comparing meat and meat alternatives: an analysis of nutrient quality in five European countries. *Public Health Nutr*. 2023;26(12):3349–58. doi: 10.1017/S136898002300194

571 Nájera Espinosa S, Hadida G, Jelmar Sietsma A, et al. Mapping the evidence of novel plant-based foods: a systematic review of nutritional, health, and environmental impacts in high-income countries. *Nutr Rev*. 2024:nuae031. doi: 10.1093/nutrit/nuae031

572 *Dietary Guidelines for Americans, 2020-2025*. 9th ed. U.S. Department of Agriculture, U.S. Department of Health and Human Services; 2020. Accessed April 24, 2025. https://www.dietaryguidelines.gov/sites/default/files/2021-03/Dietary_Guidelines_for_Americans-2020-2025.pdf

573 Whelton PK, Appel LJ, Sacco RL, et al. Sodium, blood pressure, and cardiovascular disease: further evidence supporting the American Heart Association sodium reduction recommendations. *Circulation*. 2012;126(24):2880–9. doi: 10.1161/CIR.0b013e318279acbf

574 Lindberg L, McCann RR, Smyth B, Woodside JV, Nugent AP. The environmental impact, ingredient composition, nutritional and health impact of meat alternatives: a systematic review. *Trends Food Sci Technol*. 2024;149:104483. doi: 10.1016/j.tifs.2024.104483

575 Nagra M, Tsam F, Ward S, Ur E. Animal vs plant-based meat: a hearty debate. *Can J Cardiol*. 2024;40(7):1198–209. doi: 10.1016/j.cjca.2023.11.005

576 Drewnowski A, Bruins MJ, Besselink JJF. Comparing nutrient profiles of meat and fish with plant-based alternatives: analysis of nutrients, ingredients, and fortification patterns. *Nutrients*. 2024;16(16):2725. doi: 10.3390/nu16162725

577 Messina M, Duncan AM, Glenn AJ, Mariotti F. Perspective: plant-based meat alternatives can help facilitate and maintain a lower animal to plant protein intake ratio. *Adv Nutr*. 2023;14(3):392–405. doi: 10.1016/j.advnut.2023.03.003

578 Mariotti F. Nutritional and health benefits and risks of plant-based substitute foods. *Proc Nutr Soc*. 2025;84(1):110–23. doi: 10.1017/S0029665123004767

579 Lindberg L, McCann RR, Smyth B, Woodside JV, Nugent AP. The environmental impact, ingredient composition, nutritional and health impact of meat alternatives: a systematic review. *Trends Food Sci Technol*. 2024;149:104483. doi: 10.1016/j.tifs.2024.104483

580 Plant-based meat nutrition: the facts. Good Food Institute. August 2022. Accessed May 15, 2025. https://gfi.org/resource/plant-based-meat-nutrition-facts/

581 Burger King USA nutritionals: core, regional and limited time offerings. Burger King. April 2020. Accessed May 15, 2025. http://originqa.bk.com/pdfs/nutrition.pdf

582 Rios-Mera JD, Saldaña E, Cruzado-Bravo MLM, et al. Reducing the sodium content without modifying the quality of beef burgers by adding micronized salt. *Food Res Int*. 2019;121:288–95. doi: 10.1016/j.foodres.2019.03.044

583 Tobin BD, O'Sullivan MG, Hamill RM, Kerry JP. Effect of varying salt and fat levels on the sensory quality of beef patties. *Meat Sci*. 2012;91(4):460–5. doi: 10.1016/j.meatsci.2012.02.032

584 Nájera Espinosa S, Hadida G, Jelmar Sietsma A, et al. Mapping the evidence of novel plant-based foods: a systematic review of nutritional, health, and environmental impacts in high-income countries. *Nutr Rev*. 2024:nuae031. doi: 10.1093/nutrit/nuae031

585 Nagra M, Tsam F, Ward S, Ur E. Animal vs plant-based meat: a hearty debate. *Can J Cardiol*. 2024;40(7):1198–209. doi: 10.1016/j.cjca.2023.11.005

586 Lindberg L, McCann RR, Smyth B, Woodside JV, Nugent AP. The environmental impact, ingredient composition, nutritional and health impact of meat alternatives: a systematic review. *Trends Food Sci Technol*. 2024;149:104483. doi: 10.1093/nutrit/nuae031

587 Toh DWK, Fu AS, Mehta KA, Lam NYL, Haldar S, Henry CJ. Plant-based meat analogs and their effects on cardiometabolic health: an 8-week randomized controlled trial comparing plant-based meat analogs with their corresponding animal-based foods. *Am J Clin Nutr*. 2024;119(6):1405–16. doi: 10.1016/j.ajcnut.2024.04.006

588 Toh DWK, Fu AS, Mehta KA, Lam NYL, Haldar S, Henry CJ. Plant-based meat analogs and their effects on cardiometabolic health: an 8-week randomized controlled trial comparing plant-based meat analogs with their corresponding animal-based foods. *Am J Clin Nutr*. 2024;119(6):1405–16. doi: 10.1016/j.ajcnut.2024.04.006

589 Dimsdale JE, Heeren MM. How reliable is nighttime blood pressure dipping? *Am J Hypertens*. 1998;11(5):606–9. doi: 10.1016/s0895-7061(98)00033-8

590 Parati G, Staessen JA. Day-night blood pressure variations: mechanisms, reproducibility and clinical relevance. *J Hypertens*. 2007;25(12):2377–80. doi: 10.1097/HJH.0b013e3282f2d116

591 Toh DWK, Fu AS, Mehta KA, Lam NYL, Haldar S, Henry CJ. Plant-based meat analogs and their effects on cardiometabolic health: an 8-week randomized controlled trial comparing plant-based meat analogs with their corresponding animal-based foods. *Am J Clin Nutr*. 2024;119(6):1405–16. doi: 10.1016/j.ajcnut.2024.04.006

592 Toh DWK, Fu AS, Mehta KA, Lam NYL, Haldar S, Henry CJ. Plant-based meat analogs and their effects on cardiometabolic health: an 8-week randomized controlled trial comparing plant-based meat analogs with their corresponding animal-based foods. *Am J Clin Nutr*. 2024;119(6):1405–16. doi: 10.1016/j.ajcnut.2024.04.006

593 Crimarco A, Springfield S, Petlura C, et al. A randomized crossover trial on the effect of plant-based compared with animal-based meat on trimethylamine-N-oxide and cardiovascular disease risk factors in generally healthy adults: Study With Appetizing Plantfood-Meat Eating Alternative Trial (SWAP-MEAT). *Am J Clin Nutr*. 2020;112(5):1188–99. doi: 10.1093/ajcn/nqaa203

594 Hosseinpour-Niazi S, Hadaegh F, Mirmiran P, et al. Effect of legumes in energy reduced Dietary Approaches to Stop Hypertension (DASH) diet on blood pressure among overweight and obese type 2 diabetic patients: a randomized controlled trial. *Diabetol Metab Syndr*. 2022;14(1):72. doi: 10.1186/s13098-022-00841-w

595 Astrup A, Monteiro CA. Does the concept of "ultra-processed foods" help inform dietary guidelines, beyond conventional classification systems? NO. *Am J Clin Nutr*. 2022;116(6):1482–8. doi: 10.1093/ajcn/nqac123

596 Colacino JA, Harris TR, Schecter A. Dietary intake is associated with phthalate body burden in a nationally representative sample. *Environ Health Perspect*. 2010;118(7):998–1003. doi: 10.1289/ehp.0901712

597 Milne MH, De Frond H, Rochman CM, Mallos NJ, Leonard GH, Baechler BR. Exposure of U.S. adults to microplastics from commonly-consumed proteins. *Environ Pollut*. 2024;343:123233. doi: 10.1016/j.envpol.2023.123233

598 Astrup A, Monteiro CA. Does the concept of "ultra-processed foods" help inform dietary guidelines, beyond conventional classification systems? NO. *Am J Clin Nutr*. 2022;116(6):1482–8. doi: 10.1093/ajcn/nqac123

599 Del Bo' C, Chehade L, Tucci M, Canclini F, Riso P, Martini D. Impact of substituting meats with plant-based analogues on health-related markers: a systematic review of human intervention studies. *Nutrients*. 2024;16(15):2498. doi: 10.3390/nu16152498

600 Kahleova H, Tintera J, Thieme L, et al. A plant-based meal affects thalamus perfusion differently than an energy- and macronutrient-matched conventional meal in men with type 2 diabetes, overweight/obese, and healthy men: a three-group randomized crossover study. *Clin Nutr*. 2021;40(4):1822–33. doi: 10.1016/j.clnu.2020.10.005

601 Kahleova H, Tintera J, Thieme L, et al. A plant-based meal affects thalamus perfusion differently than an energy- and macronutrient-matched conventional meal in men with type 2 diabetes, overweight/obese, and healthy men: a three-group randomized crossover study. *Clin Nutr*. 2021;40(4):1822–33. doi: 10.1016/j.clnu.2020.10.005

602 Klementova M, Thieme L, Haluzik M, et al. A plant-based meal increases gastrointestinal hormones and satiety more than an energy- and macronutrient-matched processed-meat meal in T2D, obese, and healthy men: a three-group randomized crossover study. *Nutrients*. 2019;11(1):157. doi: 10.3390/nu11010157

603 Dicken SJ, Dahm CC, Ibsen DB, et al. Food consumption by degree of food processing and risk of type 2 diabetes mellitus: a prospective cohort analysis of the European Prospective Investigation into Cancer and Nutrition (EPIC). *Lancet Reg Health Eur*. 2024;46:101043. doi: 10.1016/j.lanepe.2024.101043

604 Cherta-Murillo A, Lett AM, Frampton J, Chambers ES, Finnigan TJA, Frost GS. Effects of mycoprotein on glycaemic control and energy intake in humans: a systematic review. *Br J Nutr*. 2020;123(12):1321–32. doi: 10.1017/S0007114520000756

605 Quorn Meatless Chiqin Fillets. Quorn. Accessed May 15, 2025. https://www.quorn.us/products/quorn-meatless-chicken-fillets

606 Cherta-Murillo A, Lett AM, Frampton J, Chambers ES, Finnigan TJA, Frost GS. Effects of mycoprotein on glycaemic control and energy intake in humans: a systematic review. *Br J Nutr*. 2020;123(12):1321–32. doi: 10.1017/S0007114520000756

607 Bottin JH, Swann JR, Cropp E, et al. Mycoprotein reduces energy intake and postprandial insulin release without altering glucagon-like peptide-1 and peptide tyrosine-tyrosine concentrations in healthy overweight and obese adults: a randomised-controlled trial. *Br J Nutr*. 2016;116(2):360–74. doi: 10.1017/S0007114516001872

608 Nájera Espinosa S, Hadida G, Jelmar Sietsma A, et al. Mapping the evidence of novel plant-based foods: a systematic review of nutritional, health, and environmental impacts in high-income countries. *Nutr Rev*. 2024:nuae031. doi: 10.1093/nutrit/nuae031

609 Shapiro P, Cumbelich W. The history of *Neurospora crassa* in fermented foods. *Discov Food*. 2025;5(1):232. doi: 10.1007/s44187-025-00547-8

610 Bianchi F, Stewart C, Astbury NM, Cook B, Aveyard P, Jebb SA. Replacing Meat with Alternative Plant-based Products (RE-MAP): a randomized controlled trial of a multicomponent behavioral intervention to reduce meat consumption. *Am J Clin Nutr*. 2022;115(5):1357–66. doi: 10.1093/ajcn/nqab414

611 Crimarco A, Springfield S, Petlura C, et al. A randomized crossover trial on the effect of plant-based compared with animal-based meat on trimethylamine-N-oxide and cardiovascular disease risk factors in generally healthy adults: Study With Appetizing Plantfood-Meat Eating Alternative Trial (SWAP-MEAT). *Am J Clin Nutr*. 2020;112(5):1188–99. doi: 10.1093/ajcn/nqaa203

612 Kahleova H, Matoulek M, Malinska H, et al. Vegetarian diet improves insulin resistance and oxidative stress markers more than conventional diet in subjects with type 2 diabetes. *Diabet Med*. 2011;28(5):549–59. doi: 10.1111/j.1464-5491.2010.03209.x

613 Pham T, Knowles S, Bermingham E, et al. Plasma amino acid appearance and status of appetite following a single meal of red meat or a plant-based meat analog: a randomized crossover clinical trial. *Curr Dev Nutr*. 2022;6(5):nzac082. doi: 10.1093/cdn/nzac082

614 Fontana L, Cummings NE, Arriola Apelo SI, et al. Decreased consumption of branched-chain amino acids improves metabolic health. *Cell Rep*. 2016;16(2):520–30. doi: 10.1016/j.celrep.2016.05.092

615 Toth MJ, Poehlman ET. Sympathetic nervous system activity and resting metabolic rate in vegetarians. *Metabolism*. 1994;43(5):621–5. doi: 10.1016/0026-0495(94)90205-4

616 Montalcini T, De Bonis D, Ferro Y, et al. High vegetable fats intake is associated with high resting energy expenditure in vegetarians. *Nutrients*. 2015;7(7):5933–47. doi: 10.3390/nu7075259

617 Nájera Espinosa S, Hadida G, Jelmar Sietsma A, et al. Mapping the evidence of novel plant-based foods: a systematic review of nutritional, health, and environmental impacts in high-income countries. *Nutr Rev*. 2024:nuae031. doi: 10.1093/nutrit/nuae031

618 Toh DWK, Fu AS, Mehta KA, Lam NYL, Haldar S, Henry CJ. Plant-based meat analogs and their effects on cardiometabolic health: an 8-week randomized controlled trial comparing plant-based meat analogs with their corresponding animal-based foods. *Am J Clin Nutr*. 2024;119(6):1405–16. doi: 10.1016/j.ajcnut.2024.04.006

619 Fotouhi Ardakani A, Anjom-Shoae J, Sadeghi O, Marathe CS, Feinle-Bisset C, Horowitz M. Association between total, animal, and plant protein intake and type 2 diabetes risk in adults: a systematic review and dose-response meta-analysis of prospective cohort studies. *Clin Nutr*. 2024;43(8):1941–55. doi: 10.1016/j.clnu.2024.07.001

620 Viguiliouk E, Stewart SE, Jayalath VH, et al. Effect of replacing animal protein with plant protein on glycemic control in diabetes: a systematic review and meta-analysis of randomized controlled trials. *Nutrients*. 2015;7(12):9804–24. doi: 10.3390/nu7125509

621 Delpino FM, Figueiredo LM, Bielemann RM, et al. Ultra-processed food and risk of type 2 diabetes: a systematic review and meta-analysis of longitudinal studies. *Int J Epidemiol*. 2022;51(4):1120–41. doi: 10.1093/ije/dyab247

622 Azadbakht L, Atabak S, Esmaillzadeh A. Soy protein intake, cardiorenal indices, and C-reactive protein in type 2 diabetes with nephropathy: a longitudinal randomized clinical trial. *Diabetes Care*. 2008;31(4):648–54. doi: 10.2337/dc07-2065

623 Azadbakht L, Kimiagar M, Mehrabi Y, et al. Soy inclusion in the diet improves features of the metabolic syndrome: a randomized crossover study in postmenopausal women. *Am J Clin Nutr*. 2007;85(3):735–41. doi: 10.1093/ajcn/85.3.735

624 Jamilian M, Asemi Z. The effect of soy intake on metabolic profiles of women with gestational diabetes mellitus. *J Clin Endocrinol Metab*. 2015;100(12):4654–61. doi: 10.1210/jc.2015-3454

625 Crimarco A, Springfield S, Petlura C, et al. A randomized crossover trial on the effect of plant-based compared with animal-based meat on trimethylamine-N-oxide and cardiovascular disease risk factors in generally healthy adults: Study With Appetizing Plantfood-Meat Eating Alternative Trial (SWAP-MEAT). *Am J Clin Nutr*. 2020;112(5):1188–99. doi: 10.1093/ajcn/nqaa203

626 Toh DWK, Fu AS, Mehta KA, Lam NYL, Haldar S, Henry CJ. Plant-based meat analogs and their effects on cardiometabolic health: an 8-week randomized controlled trial comparing plant-based meat analogs with their corresponding animal-based foods. *Am J Clin Nutr*. 2024;119(6):1405–16. doi: 10.1016/j.ajcnut.2024.04.006

627 Cherta-Murillo A, Frost GS. The association of mycoprotein-based food consumption with diet quality, energy intake and non-communicable diseases' risk in the UK adult population using the National Diet and Nutrition Survey (NDNS) years 2008/2009–2016/2017: a cross-sectional study. *Br J Nutr*. 2022;127(11):1685–94. doi: 10.1017/S000711452100218X

628 Shahid M, Gaines A, Coyle D, et al. The effect of mycoprotein intake on biomarkers of human health: a systematic review and meta-analysis. *Am J Clin Nutr*. 2023;118(1):141–50. doi: 10.1016/j.ajcnut.2023.03.019

629 Cherta-Murillo A, Lett AM, Frampton J, Chambers ES, Finnigan TJA, Frost GS. Effects of mycoprotein on glycaemic control and energy intake in humans: a systematic review. *Br J Nutr*. 2020;123(12):1321–32. doi: 10.1017/S0007114520000756

630 Bottin JH, Swann JR, Cropp E, et al. Mycoprotein reduces energy intake and postprandial insulin release without altering glucagon-like peptide-1 and peptide tyrosine-tyrosine concentrations in healthy overweight and obese adults: a randomised-controlled trial. *Br J Nutr*. 2016;116(2):360–74. doi: 10.1017/S0007114516001872

631 Fryar CD, Carroll MD, Gu Q, Afful J, Ogden CL. Anthropometric reference data for children and adults: United States, 2015–2018. *Vital Health Stat 3*. 2021;(36):1–44. PMID: 33541517

632 Coelho MOC, Monteyne AJ, Dirks ML, Finnigan TJA, Stephens FB, Wall BT. Daily mycoprotein consumption for 1 week does not affect insulin sensitivity or glycaemic control but modulates the plasma lipidome in healthy adults: a randomised controlled trial. *Br J Nutr*. 2021;125(2):147–60. doi: 10.1017/S0007114520002524

633 Astrup A, Monteiro CA. Does the concept of "ultra-processed foods" help inform dietary guidelines, beyond conventional classification systems? NO. *Am J Clin Nutr*. 2022;116(6):1482–8. doi: 10.1093/ajcn/nqac123

634 Toribio-Mateas MA, Bester A, Klimenko N. Impact of plant-based meat alternatives on the gut microbiota of consumers: a real-world study. *Foods*. 2021;10(9):2040. doi: 10.3390/foods10092040

635 Farsi DN, Gallegos JL, Koutsidis G, et al. Substituting meat for mycoprotein reduces genotoxicity and increases the abundance of beneficial microbes in the gut: mycomeat, a randomised crossover control trial. *Eur J Nutr*. 2023;62(3):1479–92. doi: 10.1007/s00394-023-03088-x

636 Farsi DN, Gallegos JL, Finnigan TJA, Cheung W, Munoz JM, Commane DM. The effects of substituting red and processed meat for mycoprotein on biomarkers of cardiovascular risk in healthy volunteers: an analysis of secondary endpoints from Mycomeat. *Eur J Nutr*. 2023;62(8):3349–59. doi: 10.1007/s00394-023-03238-1

637 Crimarco A, Springfield S, Petlura C, et al. A randomized crossover trial on the effect of plant-based compared with animal-based meat on trimethylamine-N-oxide and cardiovascular disease risk factors in generally healthy adults: Study With Appetizing Plantfood-Meat Eating Alternative Trial (SWAP-MEAT). *Am J Clin Nutr*. 2020;112(5):1188–99. doi: 10.1093/ajcn/nqaa203

638 Falony G, Vieira-Silva S, Raes J. Microbiology meets big data: the case of gut microbiota-derived trimethylamine. *Annu Rev Microbiol*. 2015;69:305–21. doi: 10.1146/annurev-micro-091014-104422

639 Cleveland Clinic. TMAO takes off. *Cardiac Consult*. 2015;25(1). https://my.clevelandclinic.org/departments/heart/medical-professionals/publications/-/scassets/88d459ae7142442ba3ed0fbc6cf5c9f1.ashx

640 Spence JD, Srichaikul K, Jenkins DJA. Cardiovascular harm from egg yolk and meat: more than just cholesterol and saturated fat. *JAHA*. 2021;10(7):e017066. doi: 10.1161/JAHA.120.017066

641 Li D, Lu Y, Yuan S, et al. Gut microbiota-derived metabolite trimethylamine-N-oxide and multiple health outcomes: an umbrella review and updated meta-analysis. *Am J Clin Nutr*. 2022;116(1):230–43. doi: 10.1093/ajcn/nqac074

642 Ottiger M, Nickler M, Steuer C, et al. Gut, microbiota-dependent trimethylamine-N-oxide is associated with long-term all-cause mortality in patients with exacerbated chronic obstructive pulmonary disease. *Nutrition*. 2018;45:135–41.e1. doi: 10.1016/j.nut.2017.07.001

643 Buawangpong N, Pinyopornpanish K, Siri-Angkul N, Chattipakorn N, Chattipakorn SC. The role of trimethylamine-N-Oxide in the development of Alzheimer's disease. *J Cell Physiol*. 2022;237(3):1661–85. doi: 10.1002/jcp.30646

644 Li D, Lu Y, Yuan S, et al. Gut microbiota-derived metabolite trimethylamine-N-oxide and multiple health outcomes: an umbrella review and updated meta-analysis. *Am J Clin Nutr*. 2022;116(1):230–43. doi: 10.1093/ajcn/nqac074

645 Tang WH, Wang Z, Kennedy DJ, et al. Gut microbiota-dependent trimethylamine N-oxide (TMAO) pathway contributes to both development of renal insufficiency and mortality risk in chronic kidney disease. *Circ Res*. 2015;116(3):448–55. doi: 10.1161/CIRCRESAHA.116.305360

646 Theofilis P, Vordoni A, Kalaitzidis RG. Trimethylamine N-oxide levels in non-alcoholic fatty liver disease: a systematic review and meta-analysis. *Metabolites*. 2022;12(12):1243. doi: 10.3390/metabo12121243

647 Li D, Lu Y, Yuan S, et al. Gut microbiota-derived metabolite trimethylamine-N-oxide and multiple health outcomes: an umbrella review and updated meta-analysis. *Am J Clin Nutr*. 2022;116(1):230–43. doi: 10.1093/ajcn/nqac074

648 Zhou H, Luo Y, Zhang W, et al. Causal effect of gut-microbiota-derived metabolite trimethylamine N-oxide on Parkinson's disease: a Mendelian randomization study. *Eur J Neurol*. 2023;30(11):3451–61. doi: 10.1111/ene.15702

649 Winther SA, Rossing P. TMAO: Trimethylamine-N-oxide or time to minimize intake of animal products? *J Clin Endocrinol Metab*. 2020;105(12):dgaa428. doi: 10.1210/clinem/dgaa428

650 Martinucci I, Guidi G, Savarino EV, et al. Vegetal and animal food proteins have a different impact in the first postprandial hour of impedance-pH analysis in patients with heartburn. *Gastroenterol Res Pract*. 2018;2018:7572430.

651 Crimarco A, Landry MJ, Carter MM, Gardner CD. Assessing the effects of alternative plant-based meats v. animal meats on biomarkers of inflammation: a secondary analysis of the SWAP-MEAT randomized crossover trial. *J Nutr Sci*. 2022;11:e82. doi: 10.1017/jns.2022.84

652 Najjar RS, Moore CE, Montgomery BD. Consumption of a defined, plant-based diet reduces lipoprotein(a), inflammation, and other atherogenic lipoproteins and particles within 4 weeks. *Clin Cardiol*. 2018;41(8):1062–68. doi: 10.1002/clc.23027

653 Crimarco A, Landry MJ, Carter MM, Gardner CD. Assessing the effects of alternative plant-based meats v. animal meats on biomarkers of inflammation: a secondary analysis of the SWAP-MEAT randomized crossover trial. *J Nutr Sci*. 2022;11:e82. doi: 10.1017/jns.2022.84

654 Shivappa N, Steck SE, Hurley TG, Hussey JR, Hébert JR. Designing and developing a literature-derived, population-based dietary inflammatory index. *Public Health Nutr*. 2014;17(8):1689–96. doi: 10.1017/S1368980013002115

655 Kračmerová J, Czudková E, Koc M, et al. Postprandial inflammation is not associated with endoplasmic reticulum stress in peripheral blood mononuclear cells from healthy lean men. *Br J Nutr*. 2014;112(4):573–82. doi: 10.1017/S0007114514001093

656 Azadbakht L, Atabak S, Esmaillzadeh A. Soy protein intake, cardiorenal indices, and C-reactive protein in type 2 diabetes with nephropathy: a longitudinal randomized clinical trial. *Diabetes Care*. 2008;31(4):648–54. doi: 10.2337/dc07-2065

657　Azadbakht L, Atabak S, Esmaillzadeh A. Soy protein intake, cardiorenal indices, and C-reactive protein in type 2 diabetes with nephropathy: a longitudinal randomized clinical trial. *Diabetes Care.* 2008;31(4):648–54. doi: 10.2337/dc07-2065

658　Kaneko T, Yoshioka M, Kawahara F, et al. Effects of plant- and animal-based-protein meals for a day on serum nitric oxide and peroxynitrite levels in healthy young men. *Endocr J.* 2024;71(2):119–27. doi: 10.1507/endocrj.EJ23-0355

659　Cupisti A, Ghiadoni L, D'Alessandro C, et al. Soy protein diet improves endothelial dysfunction in renal transplant patients. *Nephrol Dial Transplant.* 2007;22(1):229–34. doi: 10.1093/ndt/gfl553

660　Cupisti A, D'Alessandro C, Ghiadoni L, Morelli E, Panichi V, Barsotti G. Effect of a soy protein diet on serum lipids of renal transplant patients. *J Ren Nutr.* 2004;14(1):31–5. doi: 10.1053/j.jrn.2003.09.007

661　Karamali M, Kashanian M, Alaeinasab S, Asemi Z. The effect of dietary soy intake on weight loss, glycaemic control, lipid profiles and biomarkers of inflammation and oxidative stress in women with polycystic ovary syndrome: a randomised clinical trial. *J Hum Nutr Diet.* 2018;31(4):533–43. doi: 10.1111/jhn.12545

662　Khoubnasabjafari M, Ansarin K, Jouyban A. Reliability of malondialdehyde as a biomarker of oxidative stress in psychological disorders. *Bioimpacts.* 2015;5(3):123–7. doi: 10.15171/bi.2015.20

663　Azadbakht L, Kimiagar M, Mehrabi Y, Esmaillzadeh A, Hu FB, Willett WC. Dietary soya intake alters plasma antioxidant status and lipid peroxidation in postmenopausal women with the metabolic syndrome. *Br J Nutr.* 2007;98(4):807–13. doi: 10.1017/S0007114507746871

664　Carlsen MH, Halvorsen BL, Holte K, et al. The total antioxidant content of more than 3,100 foods, beverages, spices, herbs and supplements used worldwide. *Nutr J.* 2010;9:3. doi: 10.1186/1475-2891-9-3

665　Malinska H, Klementová M, Kudlackova M, et al. A plant-based meal reduces postprandial oxidative and dicarbonyl stress in men with diabetes or obesity compared with an energy- and macronutrient-matched conventional meal in a randomized crossover study. *Nutr Metab.* 2021;18(1):84. doi: 10.1186/s12986-021-00609-5

666　Astrup A, Monteiro CA. Does the concept of "ultra-processed foods" help inform dietary guidelines, beyond conventional classification systems? NO. *Am J Clin Nutr.* 2022;116(6):1482–8. doi: 10.1093/ajcn/nqac123

667　Astrup A, Monteiro CA. Does the concept of "ultra-processed foods" help inform dietary guidelines, beyond conventional classification systems? NO. *Am J Clin Nutr.* 2022;116(6):1482–8. doi: 10.1093/ajcn/nqac123

668　Bryant CJ. Plant-based animal product alternatives are healthier and more environmentally sustainable than animal products. *Future Foods.* 2022;6:100174. doi: 10.1016/j.fufo.2022.100174

669　The Center for Consumer Freedom. *Synthetic Meat Spelling Bee Commercial: 30 Seconds.* YouTube. January 29, 2020. Accessed May 23, 2025. https://www.youtube.com/watch?v=jC16c_EyqP4&ab_channel=ConsumerFreedom

670　Impossible Foods. *Impossible™ Spelling Bee.* YouTube. February 2, 2020. Accessed May 23, 2025. https://www.youtube.com/watch?v=NwFRMmRyRfQ&ab_channel=ImpossibleFoods

671 Eltholth MM, Marsh VR, Van Winden S, Guitian FJ. Contamination of food products with mycobacterium avium paratuberculosis: a systematic review. *J Appl Microbiol*. 2009;107(4):1061–71. doi: 10.1111/j.1365-2672.2009.04286.x

672 Giombelli A, Gloria MB. Prevalence of *Salmonella* and *Campylobacter* on broiler chickens from farm to slaughter and efficiency of methods to remove visible fecal contamination. *J Food Prot*. 2014;77(11):1851–9. doi: 10.4315/0362-028X.JFP-14-200

673 Seo Y, Lee H, Mo C, et al. Multispectral fluorescence imaging technique for on-line inspection of fecal residues on poultry carcasses. *Sensors*. 2019;19(16):3483. doi: 10.3390/s19163483

674 Food and Drug Administration. *2021 NARMS Update: Integrated Report Summary*. August 20, 2024. Accessed May 23, 2025. https://www.fda.gov/animal-veterinary/national-antimicrobial-resistance-monitoring-system/2021-narms-update-integrated-report-summary

675 Kim MS, Lefcourt AM, Chen YR. Optimal fluorescence excitation and emission bands for detection of fecal contamination. *J Food Prot*. 2003;66(7):1198–207. doi: 10.4315/0362-028x-66.7.1198

676 Johnson J. Predictive microorgamisms as an indication of pathogen contamination. *Recip Meat Conf Proc*. 1996;49:138–43. https://meatscience.org/docs/default-source/publications-resources/rmc/1996/predictive-microorganisms-as-an-indication-of-pathogen-contamination.pdf?sfvrsn=c04fbbb3_2

677 Scallan E, Hoekstra RM, Angulo FJ, et al. Foodborne illness acquired in the United States—major pathogens. *Emerg Infect Dis*. 2011;17(1):7–15. doi: 10.3201/eid1701.p11101

678 Food and Drug Administration. *2021 NARMS Update: Integrated Report Summary*. August 20, 2024. Accessed May 23, 2025. https://www.fda.gov/animal-veterinary/national-antimicrobial-resistance-monitoring-system/2021-narms-update-integrated-report-summary

679 Scallan E, Hoekstra RM, Angulo FJ, et al. Foodborne illness acquired in the United States—major pathogens. *Emerg Infect Dis*. 2011;17(1):7–15. doi: 10.3201/eid1701.p11101

680 Food and Drug Administration. *2021 NARMS Update: Integrated Report Summary*. August 20, 2024. Accessed May 23, 2025. https://www.fda.gov/animal-veterinary/national-antimicrobial-resistance-monitoring-system/2021-narms-update-integrated-report-summary

681 Burgess F, Little CL, Allen G, Williamson K, Mitchelli RT. Prevalence of *Campylobacter*, *Salmonella*, and *Escherichia coli* on the external packaging of raw meat. *J Food Prot*. 2005;68(3):469–75. doi: 10.4315/0362-028x-68.3.469

682 Saier MH Jr, Baird SM, Reddy BL, Kopkowski PW. Eating animal products, a common cause of human diseases. *Microb Physiol*. 2022;32(5-6):146–57. doi: 10.1159/000526443

683 Chai SJ, Cole D, Nisler A, Mahon BE. Poultry: the most common food in outbreaks with known pathogens, United States, 1998–2012. *Epidemiol Infect*. 2017;145(2):316–25. doi: 10.1017/S0950268816002375

684 Batz MB, Hoffmann S, Morris JG Jr. Ranking the disease burden of 14 pathogens in food sources in the United States using attribution data from outbreak investigations and expert elicitation. *J Food Prot*. 2012;75(7):1278–91. doi: 10.4315/0362-028X.JFP-11-418

685 Jones JL, Parise ME, Fiore AE. Neglected parasitic infections in the United States: toxoplasmosis. *Am J Trop Med Hyg*. 2014;90(5):794–9. doi: 10.4269/ajtmh.13-0722

686 Guo M, Mishra A, Buchanan RL, et al. Development of dose-response models to predict the relationship for human *Toxoplasma gondii* infection associated with meat consumption. *Risk Anal*. 2016;36(5):926–38. doi: 10.1111/risa.12500

687 Wallin MT, Pretell EJ, Bustos JA, et al. Cognitive changes and quality of life in neurocysticercosis: a longitudinal study. *PLoS Negl Trop Dis*. 2012;6(1):e1493. doi: 10.1371/journal.pntd.0001493

688 Byrnes E, Shaw B, Shaw R, Madruga M, Carlan SJ. Neurocysticercosis presenting as migraine in the United States. *Am J Case Rep*. 2024;25:e943133. doi: 10.12659/AJCR.943133

689 Liu CM, Aziz M, Park DE, et al. Using source-associated mobile genetic elements to identify zoonotic extraintestinal *E. coli* infections. *One Health*. 2023;16:100518. doi: 10.1016/j.onehlt.2023.100518

690 Li P, Ji Y, Li Y, Ma Z, Pan Q. Estimating the global prevalence of hepatitis E virus in swine and pork products. *One Health*. 2021;14:100362. doi: 10.1016/j.onehlt.2021.100362

691 Saier MH Jr, Baird SM, Reddy BL, Kopkowski PW. Eating animal products, a common cause of human diseases. *Microb Physiol*. 2022;32(5-6):146–57. doi: 10.1159/000526443

692 Bobkov M, Zbinden P. Occurrence of veterinary drug residues in poultry and products thereof. A review. *Chimia*. 2018;72(10):707–12. doi: 10.2533/chimia.2018.707

693 Food and Drug Administration. *2022 Summary Report on Antimicrobials Sold or Distributed for Use in Food-Producing Animals*. December 7, 2023. Accessed May 24, 2025. https://www.fda.gov/animal-veterinary/antimicrobial-resistance/2022-summary-report-antimicrobials-sold-or-distributed-use-food-producing-animals

694 Aitken SL, Dilworth TJ, Heil EL, Nailor MD. Agricultural applications for antimicrobials. A danger to human health: an official position statement of the Society of Infectious Diseases Pharmacists. *Pharmacotherapy*. 2016;36(4):422–32. doi: 10.1002/phar.1737

695 U.S. Centers for Disease Control and Prevention. *Antibiotic Resistance Threats in the United States, 2019*. U.S. Department of Health and Human Services. Revised December 2019. Accessed May 24, 2025. https://www.cdc.gov/antimicrobial-resistance/data-research/threats/index.html

696 Mujahid S, Hansen M, Miranda R, Newsom-Stewart K, Rogers JE. Prevalence and antibiotic resistance of *Salmonella* and *Campylobacter* isolates from raw chicken breasts in retail markets in the United States and comparison to data from the plant level. *Life*. 2023;13(3):642. doi: 10.3390/life13030642

697 Ali S, Alsayeqh AF. Review of major meat-borne zoonotic bacterial pathogens. *Front Public Health*. 2022;10:1045599. doi: 10.3389/fpubh.2022.1045599

698 Cohen Stuart J, van den Munckhof T, Voets G, Scharringa J, Fluit A, Hall ML. Comparison of ESBL contamination in organic and conventional retail chicken meat. *Int J Food Microbiol*. 2012;154(3):212–4. doi: 10.1016/j.ijfoodmicro.2011.12.034

699 Bohne M, Halloran J. *Meat on Drugs*. Consumer Reports; 2012. Accessed May 24, 2025. https://advocacy.consumerreports.org/wp-content/uploads/2012/06/CR_Meat_On_Drugs_Report_06-12.pdf

700 U.S. Centers for Disease Control and Prevention. *Antibiotic Resistance Threats in the United States, 2019.* U.S. Department of Health and Human Services. Revised December 2019. Accessed May 24, 2025. https://www.cdc.gov/antimicrobial-resistance/data-research/threats/index.html

701 de Alcântara Rodrigues I, Ferrari RG, Panzenhagen PHN, Mano SB, Conte-Junior CA. Antimicrobial resistance genes in bacteria from animal-based foods. *Adv Appl Microbiol.* 2020;112:143–83. doi: 10.1016/bs.aambs.2020.03.001

702 Hassan MM, El Zowalaty ME, Lundkvist Å, et al. Residual antimicrobial agents in food originating from animals. *Trends Food Sci Technol.* 2021;111:141–50. doi: 10.1016/j.tifs.2021.01.075

703 Ji K, Kho Y, Park C, et al. Influence of water and food consumption on inadvertent antibiotics intake among general population. *Environ Res.* 2010;110(7):641–9. doi: 10.1016/j.envres.2010.06.008

704 Bacanlı M, Başaran N. Importance of antibiotic residues in animal food. *Food Chem Toxicol.* 2019;125:462–6. doi: 10.1016/j.fct.2019.01.033

705 Liu Y, Wu Y, Wu J, et al. Exposure to veterinary antibiotics via food chain disrupts gut microbiota and drives increased *Escherichia coli* virulence and drug resistance in young adults. *Pathogens.* 2022;11(9):1062. doi: 10.3390/pathogens11091062

706 Dušková M, Dorotíková K, Bartáková K, Králová M, Šedo O, Kameník J. The microbial contaminants of plant-based meat analogues from the retail market. *Int J Food Microbiol.* 2024;425:110869. doi: 10.1016/j.ijfoodmicro.2024.110869

707 Bonaldo F, Avot BJP, De Cesare A, Aarestrup FM, Otani S. Foodborne pathogen dynamics in meat and meat analogues analysed using traditional microbiology and metagenomic sequencing. *Antibiotics.* 2023;13(1):16. doi: 10.3390/antibiotics13010016

708 Liu Z, Shaposhnikov M, Zhuang S, Tu T, Wang H, Wang L. Growth and survival of common spoilage and pathogenic bacteria in ground beef and plant-based meat analogues. *Food Res Int.* 2023;164:112408. doi: 10.1016/j.foodres.2022.112408

709 Wild F, Czerny M, Janssen AM, Kole APW, Zunabovic M, Domig KJ. The evolution of a plant-based alternative to meat. From niche markets to widely accepted meat alternatives. *Agro Food Ind Hi Tech.* 2014;25(1):45–9. https://publica.fraunhofer.de/entities/publication/4d763156-ca1f-4529-bc33-d41e37e4101e

710 Vial SL, Doerscher DR, Hedberg CW, Stone WA, Whisenant SJ, Schroeder CM. Microbiological testing results of boneless and ground beef purchased for the U.S. National School Lunch Program, school years 2015 to 2018. *J Food Prot.* 2019;82(10):1761–8. doi: 10.4315/0362-028X.JFP-19-241

711 Saier MH Jr, Baird SM, Reddy BL, Kopkowski PW. Eating animal products, a common cause of human diseases. *Microb Physiol.* 2022;32(5-6):146–57. doi: 10.1159/00052644

712 Wild F, Czerny M, Janssen AM, Kole APW, Zunabovic M, Domig KJ. The evolution of a plant-based alternative to meat. From niche markets to widely accepted meat alternatives. *Agro Food Ind Hi Tech.* 2014;25(1):45–9. https://publica.fraunhofer.de/entities/publication/4d763156-ca1f-4529-bc33-d41e37e4101e

713 Kabisch J, Joswig G, Böhnlein C, Fiedler G, Franz CMAP. Microbiological status of vegan ground meat products from German retail. *J Consum Prot Food Saf.* 2024;19(1):33–40. doi: 10.1007/s00003-023-01461-w

714 Nachman KE, Smith TJ. Hormone use in food animal production: assessing potential dietary exposures and breast cancer risk. *Curr Environ Health Rep*. 2015;2(1):1–14. doi: 10.1007/s40572-014-0042-8

715 Stephany RW. Hormones in meat: different approaches in the EU and in the USA. *APMIS Suppl*. 2001;(103):S357–63. doi: 10.1111/j.1600-0463.2001.tb05787.x

716 Maruyama K, Oshima T, Ohyama K. Exposure to exogenous estrogen through intake of commercial milk produced from pregnant cows. *Pediatr Int*. 2010;52(1):33-38. doi:10.1111/j.1442-200X.2009.02890.x

717 Sehmisch S, Hammer F, Christoffel J, et al. Comparison of the phytohormones genistein, resveratrol and 8-prenylnaringenin as agents for preventing osteoporosis. *Planta Med*. 2008;74(8):794–801. doi: 10.1055/s-2008-1074550

718 Sharifi-Rad J, Quispe C, Imran M, et al. Genistein: an integrative overview of its mode of action, pharmacological properties, and health benefits. *Oxid Med Cell Longev*. 2021;2021:3268136. doi: 10.1155/2021/3268136

719 Micek A, Godos J, Brzostek T, et al. Dietary phytoestrogens and biomarkers of their intake in relation to cancer survival and recurrence: a comprehensive systematic review with meta-analysis. *Nutr Rev*. 2021;79(1):42–65. doi: 10.1093/nutrit/nuaa043

720 Boutas I, Kontogeorgi A, Dimitrakakis C, Kalantaridou SN. Soy isoflavones and breast cancer risk: a meta-analysis. *In Vivo*. 2022;36(2):556–62. doi: 10.21873/invivo.12737

721 Yager JD, Davidson NE. Estrogen carcinogenesis in breast cancer. *N Engl J Med*. 2006;354(3):270–82. doi: 10.1056/NEJMra050776

722 Micek A, Godos J, Brzostek T, et al. Dietary phytoestrogens and biomarkers of their intake in relation to cancer survival and recurrence: a comprehensive systematic review with meta-analysis. *Nutr Rev*. 2021;79(1):42–65. doi: 10.1093/nutrit/nuaa043

723 Barańska A, Kanadys W, Bogdan M, et al. The role of soy isoflavones in the prevention of bone loss in postmenopausal women: a systematic review with meta-analysis of randomized controlled trials. *J Clin Med*. 2022;11(16):4676. doi: 10.3390/jcm11164676

724 Chen MN, Lin CC, Liu CF. Efficacy of phytoestrogens for menopausal symptoms: a meta-analysis and systematic review. *Climacteric*. 2015;18(2):260–9. doi: 10.3109/13697137.2014.966241

725 Messina M, Mejia SB, Cassidy A, et al. Neither soyfoods nor isoflavones warrant classification as endocrine disruptors: a technical review of the observational and clinical data. *Crit Rev Food Sci Nutr*. 2022;62(21):5824–85. doi: 10.1080/10408398.2021.1895054

726 Reed KE, Camargo J, Hamilton-Reeves J, Kurzer M, Messina M. Neither soy nor isoflavone intake affects male reproductive hormones: an expanded and updated meta-analysis of clinical studies. *Reprod Toxicol*. 2021;100:60-67. doi: 10.1016/j.reprotox.2020.12.019

727 Bhat ZF, Morton JD, Mason SL, Bekhit AEA, Bhat HF. Technological, regulatory, and ethical aspects of in vitro meat: a future slaughter-free harvest. *Compr Rev Food Sci Food Saf*. 2019;18(4):1192–208. doi: 10.1111/1541-4337.12473

728 Hernández ÁR, Boada LD, Mendoza Z, et al. Consumption of organic meat does not diminish the carcinogenic potential associated with the intake of persistent organic pollutants (POPs). *Environ Sci Pollut Res Int*. 2017;24(5):4261–73. doi: 10.1007/s11356-015-4477-8

729 Dervilly-Pinel G, Guérin T, Minvielle B, et al. Micropollutants and chemical residues in organic and conventional meat. *Food Chem*. 2017;232:218–28. doi: 10.1016/j.foodchem.2017.04.013

730 Tressou J, Ben Abdallah N, Planche C, et al. Exposure assessment for dioxin-like PCBs intake from organic and conventional meat integrating cooking and digestion effects. *Food Chem Toxicol*. 2017;110:251–61. doi: 10.1016/j.fct.2017.10.032

731 Barbosa V, Maulvault AL, Alves RN, et al. Effects of steaming on contaminants of emerging concern levels in seafood. *Food Chem Toxicol*. 2018;118:490–504. doi: 10.1016/j.fct.2018.05.047

732 Bhat ZF, Morton JD, Mason SL, Bekhit AEA, Bhat HF. Technological, regulatory, and ethical aspects of in vitro meat: a future slaughter-free harvest. *Compr Rev Food Sci Food Saf*. 2019;18(4):1192–208. doi: 10.1111/1541-4337.12473

733 Hernández ÁR, Boada LD, Almeida-González M, et al. An estimation of the carcinogenic risk associated with the intake of multiple relevant carcinogens found in meat and charcuterie products. *Sci Total Environ*. 2015;514:33–41. doi: 10.1016/j.scitotenv.2015.01.108

734 Domingo JL, Nadal M. Carcinogenicity of consumption of red and processed meat: what about environmental contaminants? *Environ Res*. 2016;145:109–15. doi: 10.1016/j.envres.2015.11.031

735 Sasso A, Latella G. Role of heme iron in the association between red meat consumption and colorectal cancer. *Nutr Cancer*. 2018;70(8):1173–83. doi: 10.1080/01635581.2018.1521441

736 Domingo JL, Nadal M. Carcinogenicity of consumption of red and processed meat: what about environmental contaminants? *Environ Res*. 2016;145:109–15. doi: 10.1016/j.envres.2015.11.031

737 Demeyer D, Mertens B, De Smet S, Ulens M. Mechanisms linking colorectal cancer to the consumption of (processed) red meat: a review. *Crit Rev Food Sci Nutr*. 2016;56(16):2747–66. doi: 10.1080/10408398.2013.873886

738 Yang S, Dai H, Lu Y, Li R, Gao C, Pan S. Trimethylamine N-oxide promotes cell proliferation and angiogenesis in colorectal cancer. *J Immunol Res*. 2022;2022:7043856. doi: 10.1155/2022/7043856

739 Demeyer D, Mertens B, De Smet S, Ulens M. Mechanisms linking colorectal cancer to the consumption of (processed) red meat: a review. *Crit Rev Food Sci Nutr*. 2016;56(16):2747–66. doi: 10.1080/10408398.2013.873886

740 Demeyer D, Mertens B, De Smet S, Ulens M. Mechanisms linking colorectal cancer to the consumption of (processed) red meat: a review. *Crit Rev Food Sci Nutr*. 2016;56(16):2747–66. doi: 10.1080/10408398.2013.873886

741 National Cancer Institute. *Identification of Top Food Sources of Various Dietary Components*. Epidemiology and Genomics Research Program; 2010. Updated November 30, 2019. Accessed April 16, 2025. https://epi.grants.cancer.gov/diet/foodsources

742 van Vliet S, Bain JR, Muehlbauer MJ, et al. A metabolomics comparison of plant-based meat and grass-fed meat indicates large nutritional differences despite comparable Nutrition Facts panels. *Sci Rep*. 2021;11(1):13828. doi: 10.1038/s41598-021-93100-3

743 Messina M, Duncan AM, Glenn AJ, Mariotti F. Perspective: plant-based meat alternatives can help facilitate and maintain a lower animal to plant protein intake ratio. *Adv Nutr*. 2023;14(3):392–405. doi: 10.1016/j.advnut.2023.03.003

744 Ables GP, Hens JR, Nichenametla SN. Methionine restriction beyond life-span extension. *Ann N Y Acad Sci*. 2016;1363:68–79. doi: 10.1111/nyas.13014

745 Wu G, Xu J, Wang Q, et al. Methionine-restricted diet: a feasible strategy against chronic or aging-related diseases. *J Agric Food Chem*. 2023;71(1):5–19. doi: 10.1021/acs.jafc.2c05829

746 Chaturvedi S, Hoffman RM, Bertino JR. Exploiting methionine restriction for cancer treatment. *Biochem Pharmacol*. 2018;154:170–3. doi: 10.1016/j.bcp.2018.05.003

747 El Sadig R, Wu J. Are novel plant-based meat alternatives the healthier choice? *Food Res Int*. 2024;183:114184. doi: 10.1016/j.foodres.2024.114184

748 Pham T, Knowles S, Bermingham E, et al. Plasma amino acid appearance and status of appetite following a single meal of red meat or a plant-based meat analog: a randomized crossover clinical trial. *Curr Dev Nutr*. 2022;6(5):nzac082. doi: 10.1093/cdn/nzac082

749 He J, Liu H, Balamurugan S, Shao S. Fatty acids and volatile flavor compounds in commercial plant-based burgers. *J Food Sci*. 2021;86(2):293–305. doi: 10.1111/1750-3841.15594

750 Tang SN, Zuber V, Tsilidis KK. Identifying and ranking causal biochemical biomarkers for breast cancer: a Mendelian randomisation study. *BMC Med*. 2022;20(1):457.

751 Watts EL, Perez-Cornago A, Fensom GK, et al. Circulating insulin-like growth factors and risks of overall, aggressive and early-onset prostate cancer: a collaborative analysis of 20 prospective studies and Mendelian randomization analysis. *Int J Epidemiol*. 2023;52(1):71–86. doi: 10.1093/ije/dyac124

752 Allen NE, Appleby PN, Davey GK, Kaaks R, Rinaldi S, Key TJ. The associations of diet with serum insulin-like growth factor I and its main binding proteins in 292 women meat-eaters, vegetarians, and vegans. *Cancer Epidemiol Biomarkers Prev*. 2002;11(11):1441–8. PMID: 12433724

753 Fraser GE, Butler FM, Shavlik DJ, et al. Longitudinal associations between vegetarian dietary habits and site-specific cancers in the Adventist Health Study-2 North American cohort. *Am J Clin Nutr*. 2025;122(2):535–43. doi: 10.1016/j.ajcnut.2025.06.006

754 Kontessis PA, Bossinakou I, Sarika L, et al. Renal, metabolic, and hormonal responses to proteins of different origin in normotensive, nonproteinuric Type I diabetic patients. *Diabetes Care*. 1995;18(9):1233. doi: 10.2337/diacare.18.9.1233

755 Crimarco A, Springfield S, Petlura C, et al. A randomized crossover trial on the effect of plant-based compared with animal-based meat on trimethylamine-N-oxide and cardiovascular disease risk factors in generally healthy adults: Study With Appetizing Plantfood-Meat Eating Alternative Trial (SWAP-MEAT). *Am J Clin Nutr*. 2020;112(5):1188–99. doi: 10.1093/ajcn/nqaa203

756 Li Y, Ou J, Huang C, Liu F, Ou S, Zheng J. Chemistry of formation and elimination of formaldehyde in foods. *Trends Food Sci Technol*. 2023;139:104134. doi: 10.1016/j.tifs.2023.104134

757 Xi J, Chen Y. Analysis of the relationship between heterocyclic amines and the oxidation and thermal decomposition of protein using the dry heated soy protein isolate system. *LWT*. 2021;148:111738. doi: 10.1016/j.lwt.2021.111738

758 Han T, Wang T, Hou H, et al. Raw to charred: changes of precursors and intermediates and their correlation with heterocyclic amines formation in grilled lamb. *Meat Sci*. 2023;195:108999. doi: 10.1016/j.meatsci.2022.108999

759 National Center for Environmental Assessment. *Formaldehyde; CASRN 50-00-0*. U.S. Environmental Protection Agency. Accessed May 24, 2025. https://cfpub.epa.gov/ncea/iris/iris_documents/documents/subst/0419_summary.pdf

760 zur Hausen H. Red meat consumption and cancer: reasons to suspect involvement of bovine infectious factors in colorectal cancer. *Int J Cancer*. 2012;130(11):2475–83. doi: 10.1002/ijc.27413

761 Peretti A, FitzGerald PC, Bliskovsky V, Buck CB, Pastrana DV. Hamburger polyomaviruses. *J Gen Virol*. 2015;96(4):833–9. doi: 10.1099/vir.0.000033

762 de Villiers EM, Gunst K, Chakraborty D, Ernst C, Bund T, Zur Hausen H. A specific class of infectious agents isolated from bovine serum and dairy products and peritumoral colon cancer tissue. *Emerg Microbes Infect*. 2019;8(1):1205–18. doi: 10.1080/22221751.2019.1651620

763 Whitley C, Gunst K, Müller H, Funk M, Zur Hausen H, de Villiers EM. Novel replication-competent circular DNA molecules from healthy cattle serum and milk and multiple sclerosis-affected human brain tissue. *Genome Announc*. 2014;2(4):e00849-14. doi: 10.1128/genomeA.00849-14

764 Buehring GC, Shen HM, Jensen HM, Jin DL, Hudes M, Block G. Exposure to bovine leukemia virus is associated with breast cancer: a case-control study. *PLoS One*. 2015;10(9):e0134304.

765 Gao A, Kouznetsova VL, Tsigelny IF. Bovine leukemia virus relation to human breast cancer: meta-analysis. *Microb Pathog*. 2020;149:104417. doi: 10.1016/j.micpath.2020.104417

766 Song M, Garrett WS, Chan AT. Nutrients, foods, and colorectal cancer prevention. *Gastroenterol*. 2015;148(6):1244–60.e16. doi: 10.1053/j.gastro.2014.12.035

767 De Filippo C, Chioccioli S, Meriggi N, et al. Gut microbiota drives colon cancer risk associated with diet: a comparative analysis of meat-based and pesco-vegetarian diets. *Microbiome*. 2024;12(1):180. doi: 10.1186/s40168-024-01900-2

768 Wirbel J, Pyl PT, Kartal E, et al. Meta-analysis of fecal metagenomes reveals global microbial signatures that are specific for colorectal cancer. *Nat Med*. 2019;25(4):679–89. doi: 10.1038/s41591-019-0406-6

769 Dahmus JD, Kotler DL, Kastenberg DM, Kistler CA. The gut microbiome and colorectal cancer: a review of bacterial pathogenesis. *J Gastrointest Oncol*. 2018;9(4):769–77. doi: 10.21037/jgo.2018.04.07

770 Ocvirk S, O'Keefe SJD. Dietary fat, bile acid metabolism and colorectal cancer. *Semin Cancer Biol*. 2021;73:347–55. doi: 10.1016/j.semcancer.2020.10.003

771 Pimenta AI, Bernardino RM, Pereira IAC. Role of sulfidogenic members of the gut microbiota in human disease. *Adv Microb Physiol*. 2024;85:145–200. doi: 10.1016/bs.ampbs.2024.04.003

772 Lindberg L, McCann RR, Smyth B, Woodside JV, Nugent AP. The environmental impact, ingredient composition, nutritional and health impact of meat alternatives: a systematic review. *Trends Food Sci Technol.* 2024;149:104483. doi: 10.1016/j.tifs.2024.104483

773 Nájera Espinosa S, Hadida G, Jelmar Sietsma A, et al. Mapping the evidence of novel plant-based foods: a systematic review of nutritional, health, and environmental impacts in high-income countries. *Nutr Rev.* 2024:nuae031. doi: 10.1093/nutrit/nuae031

774 Yang Y, Zheng Y, Ma W, Zhang Y, Sun C, Fang Y. Meat and plant-based meat analogs: nutritional profile and in vitro digestion comparison. *Food Hydrocoll.* 2023;143:108886. doi: 10.1016/j.foodhyd.2023.108886

775 Jeyakumar A, Dissabandara L, Gopalan V. A critical overview on the biological and molecular features of red and processed meat in colorectal carcinogenesis. *J Gastroenterol.* 2017;52(4):407–18. doi: 10.1007/s00535-016-1294-x

776 Szabo Z, Koczka V, Marosvolgyi T, et al. Possible biochemical processes underlying the positive health effects of plant-based diets-a narrative review. *Nutrients.* 2021;13(8):2593. doi: 10.3390/nu13082593

777 Xu R, Wang Q, Li L. A genome-wide systems analysis reveals strong link between colorectal cancer and trimethylamine N-oxide (TMAO), a gut microbial metabolite of dietary meat and fat. *BMC Genomics.* 2015;16 Suppl 7:S4. doi: 10.1186/1471-2164-16-S7-S4

778 Crimarco A, Springfield S, Petlura C, et al. A randomized crossover trial on the effect of plant-based compared with animal-based meat on trimethylamine-N-oxide and cardiovascular disease risk factors in generally healthy adults: Study With Appetizing Plantfood-meat Eating Alternative Trial (SWAP-MEAT). *Am J Clin Nutr.* 2020;112(5):1188–99. doi: 10.1093/ajcn/nqaa203

779 Kaur H, Das C, Mande SS. *In silico* analysis of putrefaction pathways in bacteria and its implication in colorectal cancer. *Front Microbiol.* 2017;8:2166. doi: 10.3389/fmicb.2017.02166

780 Hsu YH, Huang HP, Chang HR. The uremic toxin p-cresol promotes the invasion and migration on carcinoma cells via Ras and mTOR signaling. *Toxicol In Vitro.* 2019;58:126–31. doi: 10.1016/j.tiv.2019.03.029

781 Badal BD, Fagan A, Tate V, et al. Substitution of one meat-based meal with vegetarian and vegan alternatives generates lower ammonia and alters metabolites in cirrhosis: a randomized clinical trial. *Clin Transl Gastroenterol.* 2024;15(6):e1. doi: 10.14309/ctg.0000000000000707

782 Farsi DN, Gallegos JL, Koutsidis G, et al. Substituting meat for mycoprotein reduces genotoxicity and increases the abundance of beneficial microbes in the gut: Mycomeat, a randomised crossover control trial. *Eur J Nutr.* 2023;62(3):1479–92. doi: 10.1007/s00394-023-03088-x

783 Alshannaq A, Yu JH. Occurrence, toxicity, and analysis of major mycotoxins in food. *Int J Environ Res Public Health.* 2017;14(6):632. doi: 10.3390/ijerph14060632

784 Schryvers S, Jung C, Pavicich MA, Saeger S, Lachat C, Jacxsens L. Risk ranking of mycotoxins in plant-based meat and dairy alternatives under protein transition scenarios. *Food Res Int.* 2025;200:115422. doi: 10.1016/j.foodres.2024.115422

785 Mihalache OA, Dellafiora L, Dall'Asta C. Assessing the mycotoxin-related health impact of shifting from meat-based diets to soy-based meat analogues in a model scenario based on Italian consumption data. *Expo Health*. 2023;15:661–75. https://doi.org/10.1007/s12403-022-00514-z

786 Augustin Mihalache O, Torrijos R, Dall'Asta C. Occurrence of mycotoxins in meat alternatives: dietary exposure, potential health risks, and burden of disease. *Environ Int*. 2024;185:108537. doi: 10.1016/j.envint.2024.108537

787 Augustin Mihalache O, Carbonell-Rozas L, Cutroneo S, Dall'Asta C. Multi-mycotoxin determination in plant-based meat alternatives and exposure assessment. *Food Res Int*. 2023;168:112766. doi: 10.1016/j.foodres.2023.112766

788 Gupta RS, Warren CM, Smith BM, et al. Prevalence and severity of food allergies among US Adults. *JAMA Netw Open*. 2019;2(1):e185630. doi: 10.1001/jamanetworkopen.2018.5630

789 Hoff M, Trüeb RM, Ballmer-Weber BK, Vieths S, Wuethrich B. Immediate-type hypersensitivity reaction to ingestion of mycoprotein (Quorn) in a patient allergic to molds caused by acidic ribosomal protein P2. *J Allergy Clin Immunol*. 2003;111(5):1106–10. doi: 10.1067/mai.2003.1339

790 Jacobson MF, DePorter J. Self-reported adverse reactions associated with mycoprotein (Quorn-brand) containing foods. *Ann Allergy Asthma Immunol*. 2018;120(6):626–30. doi: 10.1016/j.anai.2018.03.020

791 Finnigan TJA, Wall BT, Wilde PJ, Stephens FB, Taylor SL, Freedman MR. Mycoprotein: the future of nutritious nonmeat protein, a symposium review. *Curr Dev Nutr*. 2019;3(6):nzz021. doi: 10.1093/cdn/nzz021

792 Bartholomai BM, Ruwe KM, Thurston J, et al. Safety evaluation of Neurospora crassa mycoprotein for use as a novel meat alternative and enhancer. *Food Chem Toxicol*. 2022;168:113342. doi: 10.1016/j.fct.2022.113342

793 Gupta RS, Warren CM, Smith BM, et al. Prevalence and severity of food allergies among US adults. *JAMA Netw Open*. 2019;2(1):e185630. doi: 10.1001/jamanetworkopen.2018.5630

794 Banerjee T, Crews DC, Wesson DE, et al. Dietary acid load and chronic kidney disease among adults in the United States. *BMC Nephrol*. 2014;15:137. doi: 10.1186/1471-2369-15-137

795 Osuna-Padilla IA, Leal-Escobar G, Garza-García CA, Rodríguez-Castellanos FE. Dietary acid load: mechanisms and evidence of its health repercussions. *Nefrologia*. 2019;39(4):343–54. doi: 10.1016/j.nefro.2018.10.005

796 Wieërs MLAJ, Beynon-Cobb B, Visser WJ, Attaye I. Dietary acid load in health and disease. *Pflugers Arch*. 2024;476(4):427–43. doi: 10.1007/s00424-024-02910-7

797 Mofrad MD, Daneshzad E, Azadbakht L. Dietary acid load, kidney function and risk of chronic kidney disease: a systematic review and meta-analysis of observational studies. *Int J Vitam Nutr Res*. 2021;91(3-4):343–55. doi: 10.1024/0300-9831/a000584

798 Bahrami A, Khalesi S, Ghafouri-Taleghani F, et al. Dietary acid load and the risk of cancer: a systematic review and dose-response meta-analysis of observational studies. *Eur J Cancer Prev*. 2022;31(6):577–84. doi: 10.1097/CEJ.0000000000000748

799 Keramati M, Kheirouri S, Musazadeh V, Alizadeh M. Association of high dietary acid load with the risk of cancer: a systematic review and meta-analysis of observational studies. *Front Nutr*. 2022;9:816797. doi: 10.3389/fnut.2022.816797

800 Greger M. How to treat kidney stones with diet. NutritionFacts.org. June 12, 2015. Accessed May 27, 2025. https://nutritionfacts.org/video/how-to-treat-kidney-stones-with-diet/

801 Storz MA, Ronco AL, Hannibal L. Observational and clinical evidence that plant-based nutrition reduces dietary acid load. *J Nutr Sci*. 2022;11:e93. doi: 10.1017/jns.2022.93

802 Herter J, Huber R, Storz MA. The potential renal acid load of plant-based meat alternatives. *Eur J Clin Nutr*. 2024;78(8):732–5. doi: 10.1038/s41430-024-01434-8

803 Herter J, Huber R, Storz MA. The potential renal acid load of plant-based meat alternatives. *Eur J Clin Nutr*. 2024;78(8):732–5. doi: 10.1038/s41430-024-01434-8

804 Ward CP, Landry MJ, Cunanan KM, et al. Urinary response to consuming plant-based meat alternatives in persons with normal kidney function: the SWAP-MEAT pilot trial. *Clin J Am Soc Nephrol*. 2024;19(11):1417–25. doi: 10.2215/CJN.0000000000000532

805 Ward CP, Landry MJ, Cunanan KM, et al. Urinary response to consuming plant-based meat alternatives in persons with normal kidney function: the SWAP-MEAT pilot trial. *Clin J Am Soc Nephrol*. 2024;19(11):1417–25. doi: 10.2215/CJN.0000000000000532

806 D'Amico G, Gentile MG, Manna G, et al. Effect of vegetarian soy diet on hyperlipidaemia in nephrotic syndrome. *Lancet*. 1992;339(8802):1131–4. doi: 10.1016/0140-6736(92)90731-h

807 Azadbakht L, Atabak S, Esmaillzadeh A. Soy protein intake, cardiorenal indices, and C-reactive protein in type 2 diabetes with nephropathy: a longitudinal randomized clinical trial. *Diabetes Care*. 2008;31(4):648–54. doi: 10.2337/dc07-2065

808 Anderson JW, Blake JE, Turner J, Smith BM. Effects of soy protein on renal function and proteinuria in patients with type 2 diabetes. *Am J Clin Nutr*. 1998;68(6 Suppl):1347S–53S. doi: 10.1093/ajcn/68.6.1347S

809 Azadbakht L, Esmaillzadeh A. Soy-protein consumption and kidney-related biomarkers among type 2 diabetics: a crossover, randomized clinical trial. *J Ren Nutr*. 2009;19(6):479–86. doi: 10.1053/j.jrn.2009.06.002

810 Salomé M, Mariotti F, Nicaud MC, et al. Supplemental material for: The potential effects of meat substitution on diet quality could be high if meat substitutes are optimized for nutritional composition—a modeling study in French adults (INCA3). *Eur J Nutr*. 2022;61(4):1991–2002. doi: 10.1007/s00394-021-02781-z

811 U.S. Department of Agriculture, Agricultural Research Service. *What We Eat in America, NHANES 2017–March 2020 Prepandemic Data Tables*. 2023. Accessed June 5, 2025. https://www.ars.usda.gov/nea/bhnrc/fsrg

812 U.S. Department of Agriculture, Agricultural Research Service. *What We Eat in America, NHANES 2017–March 2020 Prepandemic Data Tables*. 2023. Accessed June 5, 2025. https://www.ars.usda.gov/nea/bhnrc/fsrg

813 Nájera Espinosa S, Hadida G, Jelmar Sietsma A, et al. Mapping the evidence of novel plant-based foods: a systematic review of nutritional, health, and environmental impacts in high-income countries. *Nutr Rev*. 2024:nuae031. doi: 10.1093/nutrit/nuae031

814 Institute of Medicine (U.S.). *Dietary Reference Intakes: Proposed Definition of Dietary Fiber.* National Academies Press; 2001.

815 Nájera Espinosa S, Hadida G, Jelmar Sietsma A, et al. Mapping the evidence of novel plant-based foods: a systematic review of nutritional, health, and environmental impacts in high-income countries. *Nutr Rev.* 2024:nuae031. doi: 10.1093/nutrit/nuae031

816 Mariotti F. Nutritional and health benefits and risks of plant-based substitute foods. *Proc Nutr Soc.* 2025;84(1):110–23. doi: 10.1017/S0029665123004767

817 U.S. Department of Agriculture, Agricultural Research Service. *What We Eat in America, NHANES 2017–March 2020 Prepandemic Data Tables.* 2023. Accessed June 5, 2025. https://www.ars.usda.gov/nea/bhnrc/fsrg

818 Rizzo NS, Jaceldo-Siegl K, Sabate J, Fraser GE. Nutrient profiles of vegetarian and nonvegetarian dietary patterns. *J Acad Nutr Diet.* 2013;113(12):1610–9.

819 Institute of Medicine. *Dietary Reference Intakes: The Essential Guide to Nutrient Requirements.* The National Academies Press; 2006. https://doi.org/10.17226/11537

820 Nájera Espinosa S, Hadida G, Jelmar Sietsma A, et al. Mapping the evidence of novel plant-based foods: a systematic review of nutritional, health, and environmental impacts in high-income countries. *Nutr Rev.* 2024:nuae031. doi: 10.1093/nutrit/nuae031

821 van Vliet S, Bain JR, Muehlbauer MJ, et al. A metabolomics comparison of plant-based meat and grass-fed meat indicates large nutritional differences despite comparable nutrition facts panels. *Sci Rep.* 2021;11(1):13828. doi: 10.1038/s41598-021-93100-3

822 Curtain F, Grafenauer S. Plant-based meat substitutes in the flexitarian age: an audit of products on supermarket shelves. *Nutrients.* 2019;11(11):2603. doi: 10.3390/nu11112603

823 Neuhofer ZT, Lusk JL. Most plant-based meat alternative buyers also buy meat: an analysis of household demographics, habit formation, and buying behavior among meat alternative buyers. *Sci Rep.* 2022;12(1):13062. doi: 10.1038/s41598-022-16996-5

824 U.S. Department of Agriculture, Agricultural Research Service. *What We Eat in America, NHANES 2017–March 2020 Prepandemic Data Tables.* 2023. Accessed June 5, 2025. https://www.ars.usda.gov/nea/bhnrc/fsrg

825 Vatanparast H, Islam N, Shafiee M, Ramdath DD. Increasing plant-based meat alternatives and decreasing red and processed meat in the diet differentially affect the diet quality and nutrient intakes of Canadians. *Nutrients.* 2020;12(7):2034. doi: 10.3390/nu12072034

826 U.S. Department of Agriculture, Agricultural Research Service. *What We Eat in America, NHANES 2017–March 2020 Prepandemic Data Tables.* 2023. Accessed May 24, 2025. https://www.ars.usda.gov/nea/bhnrc/fsrg

827 Lindberg L, McCann RR, Smyth B, Woodside JV, Nugent AP. The environmental impact, ingredient composition, nutritional and health impact of meat alternatives: a systematic review. *Trends Food Sci Technol.* 2024;149:104483. doi: 10.1016/j.tifs.2024.104483

828 Latunde-Dada GO, Kajarabille N, Rose S, et al. Content and availability of minerals in plant-based burgers compared with a meat burger. *Nutrients.* 2023;15(12):2732. doi: 10.3390/nu15122732

829 U.S. Department of Agriculture, Agricultural Research Service. *What We Eat in America, NHANES 2017–March 2020 Prepandemic Data Tables.* 2023. Accessed June 5, 2025. https://www.ars.usda.gov/nea/bhnrc/fsrg

830 Harnack L, Mork S, Valluri S, et al. Nutrient composition of a selection of plant-based ground beef alternative products available in the United States. *J Acad Nutr Diet.* 2021;121(12):2401–8.e12. doi: 10.1016/j.jand.2021.05.002

831 Pointke M, Pawelzik E. Plant-based alternative products: are they healthy alternatives? Micro- and macronutrients and nutritional scoring. *Nutrients.* 2022;14(3):601. doi: 10.3390/nu14030601

832 Bryngelsson S, Moshtaghian H, Bianchi M, Hallström E. Nutritional assessment of plant-based meat analogues on the Swedish market. *Int J Food Sci Nutr.* 2022;73(7):889–901. doi: 10.1080/09637486.2022.2078286

833 van Vliet S, Bain JR, Muehlbauer MJ, et al. A metabolomics comparison of plant-based meat and grass-fed meat indicates large nutritional differences despite comparable Nutrition Facts panels. *Sci Rep.* 2021;11(1):13828. doi: 10.1038/s41598-021-93100-3

834 Borén J, Chapman MJ, Krauss RM, et al. Low-density lipoproteins cause atherosclerotic cardiovascular disease: pathophysiological, genetic, and therapeutic insights: a consensus statement from the European Atherosclerosis Society Consensus Panel. *Eur Heart J.* 2020;41(24):2313–30. doi: 10.1093/eurheartj/ehz962

835 Atar D, Jukema JW, Molemans B, et al. New cardiovascular prevention guidelines: how to optimally manage dyslipidaemia and cardiovascular risk in 2021 in patients needing secondary prevention? *Atherosclerosis.* 2021;319:51–61. doi: 10.1016/j.atherosclerosis.2020.12.013

836 Mhaimeed O, Burney ZA, Schott SL, Kohli P, Marvel FA, Martin SS. The importance of LDL-C lowering in atherosclerotic cardiovascular disease prevention: lower for longer is better. *Am J Prev Cardiol.* 2024;18:100649. doi: 10.1016/j.ajpc.2024.100649

837 Fernández-Friera L, Fuster V, López-Melgar B, et al. Normal LDL-cholesterol levels are associated with subclinical atherosclerosis in the absence of risk factors. *J Am Coll Cardiol.* 2017;70(24):2979–91. doi: 10.1016/j.jacc.2017.10.024

838 Poli A, Catapano AL, Corsini A, et al. LDL-cholesterol control in the primary prevention of cardiovascular diseases: an expert opinion for clinicians and health professionals. *Nutr Metab Cardiovasc Dis.* 2023;33(2):245–57. doi: 10.1016/j.numecd.2022.10.001

839 Borén J, Chapman MJ, Krauss RM, et al. Low-density lipoproteins cause atherosclerotic cardiovascular disease: pathophysiological, genetic, and therapeutic insights: a consensus statement from the European Atherosclerosis Society Consensus Panel. *Eur Heart J.* 2020;41(24):2313–30. doi: 10.1093/eurheartj/ehz962

840 Trumbo PR, Shimakawa T. Tolerable upper intake levels for trans fat, saturated fat, and cholesterol. *Nutr Rev.* 2011;69(5):270–8. doi: 10.1111/j.1753-4887.2011.00389.x

841 Harnack LJ, Reese MM, Johnson AJ. Are plant-based meat alternative products healthier than the animal meats they mimic? *Nutr Today.* 2022;57(4):195–9. doi: 10.1097/NT.0000000000000553

842 Food and Drug Administration. Revocation of uses of partially hydrogenated oils in foods. *Fed Regist.* 2023;88(152):53764–74.

843 Revealing trans fats. *FDA Consumer.* 2003;37(5):20–6.

844 He J, Liu H, Balamurugan S, Shao S. Fatty acids and volatile flavor compounds in commercial plant-based burgers. *J Food Sci.* 2021;86(2):293–305. doi: 10.1111/1750-3841.15594

845 US dietary guidelines remove dietary cholesterol limit. Egg Info. August 1, 2016. Accessed May 30, 2025. https://www.egginfo.co.uk/news/us-dietary-guidelines-remove-dietary-cholesterol-limit

846 U.S. Department of Health and Human Services; U.S. Department of Agriculture. *Dietary Guidelines for Americans, 2015–2020*. 8th ed. December 2015. Accessed May 24, 2025. https://health.gov/sites/default/files/2019-09/2015-2020_Dietary_Guidelines.pdf

847 U.S. Department of Health and Human Services; U.S. Department of Agriculture. *Dietary Guidelines for Americans, 2020–2025*. 9th ed. December 2020. Accessed May 24, 2025. https://www.dietaryguidelines.gov/sites/default/files/2021-03/Dietary_Guidelines_for_Americans-2020-2025.pdf

848 Grundy SM. Does dietary cholesterol matter? *Curr Atheroscler Rep*. 2016;18(11):68. doi: 10.1007/s11883-016-0615-0

849 Harnack LJ, Reese MM, Johnson AJ. Are plant-based meat alternative products healthier than the animal meats they mimic? *Nutr Today*. 2022;57(4):195–9. doi: 10.1097/NT.0000000000000553

850 Mariotti F. Nutritional and health benefits and risks of plant-based substitute foods. *Proc Nutr Soc*. 2025;84(1):110–23. doi: 10.1017/S0029665123004767

851 Harnack L, Mork S, Valluri S, et al. Nutrient composition of a selection of plant-based ground beef alternative products available in the United States. *J Acad Nutr Diet*. 2021;121(12):2401–8.e12. doi: 10.1016/j.jand.2021.05.002

852 Popular and versatile- ground beef reigns! Cattlemen's Beef Board and National Cattlemen's Beef Association. April 11, 2019. Accessed May 30, 2025. https://www.beefitswhatsfordinner.com/retail/sales-data-shopper-insights/ground-beef-sales

853 Nájera Espinosa S, Hadida G, Jelmar Sietsma A, et al. Mapping the evidence of novel plant-based foods: a systematic review of nutritional, health, and environmental impacts in high-income countries. *Nutr Rev*. 2024:nuae031. doi: 10.1093/nutrit/nuae031

854 Nájera Espinosa S, Hadida G, Jelmar Sietsma A, et al. Mapping the evidence of novel plant-based foods: a systematic review of nutritional, health, and environmental impacts in high-income countries. *Nutr Rev*. 2024:nuae031. doi: 10.1093/nutrit/nuae031

855 Crimarco A, Springfield S, Petlura C, et al. A randomized crossover trial on the effect of plant-based compared with animal-based meat on trimethylamine-N-oxide and cardiovascular disease risk factors in generally healthy adults: Study With Appetizing Plantfood-Meat Eating Alternative Trial (SWAP-MEAT). *Am J Clin Nutr*. 2020;112(5):1188–99. doi: 10.1093/ajcn/nqaa203

856 Bianchi F, Stewart C, Astbury NM, Cook B, Aveyard P, Jebb SA. Replacing meat with alternative plant-based products (RE-MAP): a randomized controlled trial of a multicomponent behavioral intervention to reduce meat consumption. *Am J Clin Nutr*. 2022;115(5):1357–66. doi: 10.1093/ajcn/nqab414

857 Azadbakht L, Kimiagar M, Mehrabi Y, et al. Soy inclusion in the diet improves features of the metabolic syndrome: a randomized crossover study in postmenopausal women. *Am J Clin Nutr*. 2007;85(3):735–41. doi: 10.1093/ajcn/85.3.735

858 Sirtori CR, Agradi E, Conti F, Mantero O, Gatti E. Soybean-protein diet in the treatment of type-II hyperlipoproteinaemia. *Lancet*. 1977;1(8006):275–7. doi: 10.1016/s0140-6736(77)91823-2

859 Turnbull WH, Leeds AR, Edwards GD. Effect of mycoprotein on blood lipids. *Am J Clin Nutr*. 1990;52(4):646–50. doi: 10.1093/ajcn/52.4.646

860 Farsi DN, Gallegos JL, Finnigan TJA, Cheung W, Munoz JM, Commane DM. The effects of substituting red and processed meat for mycoprotein on biomarkers of cardiovascular risk in healthy volunteers: an analysis of secondary endpoints from Mycomeat. *Eur J Nutr*. 2023;62(8):3349–59. doi: 10.1007/s00394-023-03238-1

861 Gibbs J, Leung GK. The effect of plant-based and mycoprotein-based meat substitute consumption on cardiometabolic risk factors: a systematic review and meta-analysis of controlled intervention trials. *Dietetics*. 2023;2(1):104–22. doi: 10.3390/dietetics2010009

862 Ference BA, Ginsberg HN, Graham I, et al. Low-density lipoproteins cause atherosclerotic cardiovascular disease. 1. Evidence from genetic, epidemiologic, and clinical studies. A consensus statement from the European Atherosclerosis Society Consensus Panel. *Eur Heart J*. 2017;38(32):2459–72. doi: 10.1093/eurheartj/ehx144

863 Wang N, Fulcher J, Abeysuriya N, et al. Intensive LDL cholesterol-lowering treatment beyond current recommendations for the prevention of major vascular events: a systematic review and meta-analysis of randomised trials including 327,037 participants. *Lancet Diabetes Endocrinol*. 2020;8(1):36–49. doi: 10.1016/S2213-8587(19)30388-2

864 Azadbakht L, Atabak S, Esmaillzadeh A. Soy protein intake, cardiorenal indices, and C-reactive protein in type 2 diabetes with nephropathy: a longitudinal randomized clinical trial. *Diabetes Care*. 2008;31(4):648–54. doi: 10.2337/dc07-2065

865 Ference BA, Ginsberg HN, Graham I, et al. Low-density lipoproteins cause atherosclerotic cardiovascular disease. 1. Evidence from genetic, epidemiologic, and clinical studies. A consensus statement from the European Atherosclerosis Society Consensus Panel. *Eur Heart J*. 2017;38(32):2459–72. doi: 10.1093/eurheartj/ehx144

866 Martin SS, Aday AW, Almarzooq ZI, et al. 2024 heart disease and stroke statistics: a report of US and global data from the American Heart Association. *Circulation*. 2024;149(8):e347–913. doi: 10.1161/CIR.0000000000001209.

867 Petersen T, Hirsch S. Comparing meat and meat alternatives: an analysis of nutrient quality in five European countries. *Public Health Nutr*. 2023;26(12):3349–58. doi: 10.1017/S1368980023001945

868 Maki KC, Van Elswyk ME, Alexander DD, Rains TM, Sohn EL, McNeill S. A meta-analysis of randomized controlled trials that compare the lipid effects of beef versus poultry and/or fish consumption. *J Clin Lipidol*. 2012;6(4):352–61. doi: 10.1016/j.jacl.2012.01.001

869 Guasch-Ferré M, Satija A, Blondin SA, et al. Meta-analysis of randomized controlled trials of red meat consumption in comparison with various comparison diets on cardiovascular risk factors. *Circulation*. 2019;139(15):1828–45. doi: 10.1161/CIRCULATIONAHA.118.035225

870 Nájera Espinosa S, Hadida G, Jelmar Sietsma A, et al. Mapping the evidence of novel plant-based foods: a systematic review of nutritional, health, and environmental impacts in high-income countries. *Nutr Rev*. 2024:nuae031. doi: 10.1093/nutrit/nuae031

871 Toh DWK, Fu AS, Mehta KA, Lam NYL, Haldar S, Henry CJ. Plant-based meat analogs and their effects on cardiometabolic health: an 8-week randomized controlled trial comparing plant-based meat analogs with their corresponding animal-based foods. *Am J Clin Nutr*. 2024;119(6):1405–16. doi: 10.1016/j.ajcnut.2024.04.006

872 Turnbull WH, Leeds AR, Edwards GD. Effect of mycoprotein on blood lipids. *Am J Clin Nutr*. 1990;52(4):646–50. doi: 10.1093/ajcn/52.4.646

873 Turnbull WH, Leeds AR, Edwards GD. Effect of mycoprotein on blood lipids. *Am J Clin Nutr*. 1990;52(4):646–50. doi: 10.1093/ajcn/52.4.646

874 Turnbull WH, Leeds AR, Edwards GD. Effect of mycoprotein on blood lipids. *Am J Clin Nutr*. 1990;52(4):646–50. doi: 10.1093/ajcn/52.4.646

875 Ghavami A, Ziaei R, Talebi S, et al. Soluble fiber supplementation and serum lipid profile: a systematic review and dose-response meta-analysis of randomized controlled trials. *Adv Nutr*. 2023;14(3):465–74. doi: 10.1016/j.advnut.2023.01.005

876 Azadbakht L, Atabak S, Esmaillzadeh A. Soy protein intake, cardiorenal indices, and C-reactive protein in type 2 diabetes with nephropathy: a longitudinal randomized clinical trial. *Diabetes Care*. 2008;31(4):648–54. doi: 10.2337/dc07-2065

877 Nagra M, Tsam F, Ward S, Ur E. Animal vs plant-based meat: a hearty debate. *Can J Cardiol*. 2024;40(7):1198–209. doi: 10.1016/j.cjca.2023.11.005

878 Grundy SM. Does dietary cholesterol matter? *Curr Atheroscler Rep*. 2016;18(11):68. doi: 10.1007/s11883-016-0615-0

879 Carroll KK, Giovannetti PM, Huff MW, Moase O, Roberts DC, Wolfe BM. Hypocholesterolemic effect of substituting soybean protein for animal protein in the diet of healthy young women. *Am J Clin Nutr*. 1978;31(8):1312–21. doi: 10.1093/ajcn/31.8.1312

880 Carroll KK, Hamilton RMG. Effects of dietary protein and carbohydrate on plasma cholesterol levels in relation to atherosclerosis. *J Food Sci*. 1975;40(1):18–23. doi: 10.1111/j.1365-2621.1975.tb03726.x

881 Bergeron N, Chiu S, Williams PT, M King S, Krauss RM. Effects of red meat, white meat, and nonmeat protein sources on atherogenic lipoprotein measures in the context of low compared with high saturated fat intake: a randomized controlled trial. *Am J Clin Nutr*. 2019;110(1):24–33. doi: 10.1093/ajcn/nqz035

882 Bergeron N, Chiu S, Williams PT, M King S, Krauss RM. Effects of red meat, white meat, and nonmeat protein sources on atherogenic lipoprotein measures in the context of low compared with high saturated fat intake: a randomized controlled trial. *Am J Clin Nutr*. 2019;110(1):24–33. doi: 10.1093/ajcn/nqz035

883 Bergeron N, Chiu S, Williams PT, M King S, Krauss RM. Effects of red meat, white meat, and nonmeat protein sources on atherogenic lipoprotein measures in the context of low compared with high saturated fat intake: a randomized controlled trial. *Am J Clin Nutr*. 2019;110(1):24–33. doi: 10.1093/ajcn/nqz035

884 Bergeron N, Chiu S, Williams PT, M King S, Krauss RM. Effects of red meat, white meat, and nonmeat protein sources on atherogenic lipoprotein measures in the context of low compared with high saturated fat intake: a randomized controlled trial. *Am J Clin Nutr*. 2019;110(1):24–33. doi: 10.1093/ajcn/nqz035

885 Vincent MJ, Allen B, Palacios OM, Haber LT, Maki KC. Meta-regression analysis of the effects of dietary cholesterol intake on LDL and HDL cholesterol. *Am J Clin Nutr*. 2019;109(1):7–16. doi: 10.1093/ajcn/nqy273

886 Li SS, Blanco Mejia S, Lytvyn L, et al. Effect of plant protein on blood lipids: a systematic review and meta-analysis of randomized controlled trials. *J Am Heart Assoc*. 2017;6(12):e006659. doi: 10.1161/JAHA.117.006659

887 Kumar P, Chatli MK, Mehta N, Singh P, Malav OP, Verma AK. Meat analogues: health promising sustainable meat substitutes. *Crit Rev Food Sci Nutr*. 2017;57(5):923–32. doi: 10.1080/10408398.2014.939739

888 Nagra M, Tsam F, Ward S, Ur E. Animal vs plant-based meat: a hearty debate. *Can J Cardiol*. 2024;40(7):1198–209. doi: 10.1016/j.cjca.2023.11.005

889 Sasso A, Latella G. Role of heme iron in the association between red meat consumption and colorectal cancer. *Nutr Cancer*. 2018;70(8):1173–83. doi: 10.1080/01635581.2018.1521441

890 De Smet S, Van Hecke T. Meat products in human nutrition and health—about hazards and risks. *Meat Sci*. 2024;218:109628. doi: 10.1016/j.meatsci.2024

891 Norat T, Scoccianti C, Boutron-Ruault MC, et al. European Code against Cancer 4th edition: diet and cancer. *Cancer Epidemiol*. 2015;39 Suppl 1:S56–66. doi: 10.1016/j.canep.2014.12.016

892 American Institute for Cancer Research. *Facts About Red Meat & Processed Meat*. Accessed June 2, 2025. https://store.aicr.org/products/facts-about-red-meat-and-processed-meats

893 Harvard University, T.H. Chan School of Public Health. *Healthy Eating Plate*. 2011. Updated January 2023. Accessed June 2, 2025. https://nutritionsource.hsph.harvard.edu/healthy-eating-plate/

894 Crowe W, Elliott CT, Green BD. A review of the *in vivo* evidence investigating the role of nitrite exposure from processed meat consumption in the development of colorectal cancer. *Nutrients*. 2019;11(11):2673. doi: 10.3390/nu11112673

895 Memorial Sloan Kettering Cancer Center. *Tips for Healthy Eating*. Updated May 16, 2022. Accessed June 2, 2025. https://www.mskcc.org/cancer-care/patient-education/tips-healthy-eating

896 University of Texas, MD Anderson Cancer Center. Processed meat and cancer: what you need to know. August 1, 2025. Accessed October 11, 2025. https://www.mdanderson.org/cancerwise/processed-meat-and-cancer-what-you-need-to-know.h00-159778812.html

897 Lescinsky H, Afshin A, Ashbaugh C, et al. Health effects associated with consumption of unprocessed red meat: a burden of proof study. *Nat Med*. 2022;28(10):2075–82. doi: 10.1038/s41591-022-01968-z

898 Kennedy J, Alexander P, Taillie LS, Jaacks LM. Estimated effects of reductions in processed meat consumption and unprocessed red meat consumption on occurrences of type 2 diabetes, cardiovascular disease, colorectal cancer, and mortality in the USA: a microsimulation study. *Lancet Planet Health*. 2024;8(7):e441–51. doi: 10.1016/S2542-5196(24)00118-9

899 GBD 2021 US Burden of Disease Collaborators. The burden of diseases, injuries, and risk factors by state in the USA, 1990-2021: a systematic analysis for the Global Burden of Disease Study 2021. *Lancet*. 2024;404(10469):2314–40. doi: 10.1016/S0140-6736(24)01446-6

900 Global Health Metrics. Diet high in processed meat—level 3 risk. *Lancet*. October 17, 2020. Accessed October 11, 2025. https://www.thelancet.com/pb-assets/Lancet/gbd/summaries/risks/diet-processed-meat.pdf

901   Global Health Metrics. Diet high in red meat—Level 3 risk. *Lancet.* October 17, 2020. Accessed October 11, 2025. https://www.thelancet.com/pb-assets/Lancet/gbd/summaries/risks/diet-red-meat.pdf

902   Grosso G, La Vignera S, Condorelli RA, et al. Total, red and processed meat consumption and human health: an umbrella review of observational studies. *Int J Food Sci Nutr.* 2022;73(6):726–37. doi: 10.1080/09637486.2022.2050996

903   Ritchie H, Reay DS, Higgins P. Potential of meat substitutes for climate change mitigation and improved human health in high-income markets. *Front Sustain Food Syst.* 2018;2:16. doi: 10.3389/fsufs.2018.00016

904   Reynolds AN, Mhurchu CN, Kok ZY, Cleghorn C. The neglected potential of red and processed meat replacement with alternative protein sources: simulation modelling and systematic review. *EClinicalMedicine.* 2022;56:101774. doi: 10.1016/j.eclinm.2022.101774

905   Nájera Espinosa S, Hadida G, Jelmar Sietsma A, et al. Mapping the evidence of novel plant-based foods: a systematic review of nutritional, health, and environmental impacts in high-income countries. *Nutr Rev.* 2024:nuae031. doi: 10.1093/nutrit/nuae031

906   UBS Global Wealth Management, Chief Investment Office. *The Food Revolution – The Future of Food and the Challenges We Face.* UBS. July 29, 2019. Accessed June 3, 2025. https://web.archive.org/web/20211108102410/https://www.ubs.com/global/en/wealth-management/insights/chief-investment-office/sustainable-investing/2019/food-revolution.html

907   Rios-Mera JD, Saldaña E, Cruzado-Bravo MLM, et al. Reducing the sodium content without modifying the quality of beef burgers by adding micronized salt. *Food Res Int.* 2019;121:288–95. doi: 10.1016/j.foodres.2019.03.044

908   Beyond Meat unveils its Beyond IV platform, the fourth generation of the Beyond Burger and Beyond Beef. BeyondMeat.com. February 21, 2024. Accessed June 3, 2025. https://www.beyondmeat.com/en-US/press/beyond-meat-unveils-its-beyond-iv-platform-the-fourth-generation-of-the-beyond-burger-and-beyond-beef

909   Impossible Beef Lite. Impossiblefoods.com. Accessed June 3, 2025. https://impossiblefoods.com/beef/plant-based-impossible-beef-lite

910   U.S. Department of Health and Human Services; U.S. Department of Agriculture. *Dietary Guidelines for Americans, 2020–2025.* 9th ed. December 2020. Accessed May 24, 2025. https://www.dietaryguidelines.gov/sites/default/files/2021-03/Dietary_Guidelines_for_Americans-2020-2025.pdf

911   Messina MJ, Sievenpiper JL, Williamson P, Kiel J, Erdman JW Jr. Ultra-processed foods: a concept in need of revision to avoid targeting healthful and sustainable plant-based foods. *Public Health Nutr.* 2023;26(7):1390–1. doi: 10.1017/S1368980023000617

912   Messina M, Sievenpiper JL, Williamson P, Kiel J, Erdman JW. Perspective: soy-based meat and dairy alternatives, despite classification as ultra-processed foods, deliver high-quality nutrition on par with unprocessed or minimally processed animal-based counterparts. *Adv Nutr.* 2022;13(3):726–38. doi: 10.1093/advances/nmac026

913   Bestari FF, Andarwulan N, Palupi E. Synthesis of effect sizes on dose response from ultra-processed food consumption against various noncommunicable diseases. *Foods.* 2023;12(24):4457. doi: 10.3390/foods12244457

914   Yuan L, Hu H, Li T, et al. Dose-response meta-analysis of ultra-processed food with the risk of cardiovascular events and all-cause mortality: evidence from prospective cohort studies. *Food Funct.* 2023;14(6):2586–96. doi: 10.1039/d2fo02628g

915 Juul F, Vaidean G, Lin Y, Deierlein AL, Parekh N. Ultra-processed foods and incident cardiovascular disease in the Framingham Offspring Study. *J Am Coll Cardiol.* 2021;77(12):1520–31. doi: 10.1016/j.jacc.2021.01.047

916 Zhong GC, Gu HT, Peng Y, et al. Association of ultra-processed food consumption with cardiovascular mortality in the US population: long-term results from a large prospective multicenter study. *Int J Behav Nutr Phys Act.* 2021;18(1):21. doi: 10.1186/s12966-021-01081-3

917 Zhong GC, Gu HT, Peng Y, et al. Supplementary material for: Association of ultra-processed food consumption with cardiovascular mortality in the US population: long-term results from a large prospective multicenter study. *Int J Behav Nutr Phys Act.* 2021;18(1):21. doi: 10.1186/s12966-021-01081-3

918 Mendoza K, Smith-Warner SA, Rossato SL, et al. Ultra-processed foods and cardiovascular disease: analysis of three large US prospective cohorts and a systematic review and meta-analysis of prospective cohort studies. *Lancet Reg Health Am.* 2024;37:100859. doi: 10.1016/j.lana.2024.100859

919 Rivera N, Du S, Bernard L, Kim H, Matsushita K, Rebholz CM. Ultra-processed food consumption and risk of incident hypertension in US middle-aged adults. *J Am Heart Assoc.* 2024;13(17):e035189. doi: 10.1161/JAHA.124.035189

920 Mendoza K, Smith-Warner SA, Rossato SL, et al. Ultra-processed foods and cardiovascular disease: analysis of three large US prospective cohorts and a systematic review and meta-analysis of prospective cohort studies. *Lancet Reg Health Am.* 2024;37:100859. doi: 10.1016/j.lana.2024.100859

921 Mendoza K, Smith-Warner SA, Rossato SL, et al. Ultra-processed foods and cardiovascular disease: analysis of three large US prospective cohorts and a systematic review and meta-analysis of prospective cohort studies. *Lancet Reg Health Am.* 2024;37:100859. doi: 10.1016/j.lana.2024.100859

922 Kliemann N, Rauber F, Bertazzi Levy R, et al. Food processing and cancer risk in Europe: results from the prospective EPIC cohort study. *Lancet Planet Health.* 2023;7(3):e219–32. doi: 10.1016/S2542-5196(23)00021-9

923 Wang L, Du M, Wang K, et al. Association of ultra-processed food consumption with colorectal cancer risk among men and women: results from three prospective US cohort studies. *BMJ.* 2022;378:e068921. doi: 10.1136/bmj-2021-068921

924 Zhong GC, Zhu Q, Cai D, et al. Ultra-processed food consumption and the risk of pancreatic cancer in the prostate, lung, colorectal and ovarian cancer screening trial. *Int J Cancer.* 2023;152(5):835–44. doi: 10.1002/ijc.34290

925 Chen Z, Khandpur N, Desjardins C, et al. Ultra-processed food consumption and risk of type 2 diabetes: three large prospective U.S. cohort studies. *Diabetes Care.* 2023;46(7):1335–44. doi: 10.2337/dc22-1993

926 Fang Z, Rossato SL, Hang D, et al. Association of ultra-processed food consumption with all cause and cause specific mortality: population based cohort study. *BMJ.* 2024;385:e078476. doi: 10.1136/bmj-2023-078476

927 Fang Z, Rossato SL, Hang D, et al. Association of ultra-processed food consumption with all cause and cause specific mortality: population based cohort study. *BMJ.* 2024;385:e078476. doi: 10.1136/bmj-2023-078476

oly.

928 Taneri PE, Wehrli F, Roa-Díaz ZM, et al. Association between ultra-processed food intake and all-cause mortality: a systematic review and meta-analysis. *Am J Epidemiol*. 2022;191(7):1323–35. doi: 10.1093/aje/kwac039

929 Taneri PE, Wehrli F, Roa-Díaz ZM, et al. Association between ultra-processed food intake and all-cause mortality: a systematic review and meta-analysis. *Am J Epidemiol*. 2022;191(7):1323–35. doi: 10.1093/aje/kwac039

930 Fang Z, Rossato SL, Hang D, et al. Association of ultra-processed food consumption with all cause and cause specific mortality: population based cohort study. *BMJ*. 2024;385:e078476. doi: 10.1136/bmj-2023-078476

931 Orlich MJ, Sabaté J, Mashchak A, et al. Ultra-processed food intake and animal-based food intake and mortality in the Adventist Health Study-2. *Am J Clin Nutr*. 2022;115(6):1589–601. doi: 10.1093/ajcn/nqac043

932 Rauber F, Laura da Costa Louzada M, Chang K, et al. Implications of food ultra-processing on cardiovascular risk considering plant origin foods: an analysis of the UK biobank cohort. *Lancet Reg Health Eur*. 2024;43:100948. doi: 10.1016/j.lanepe.2024.100948

933 Clay X. The hidden health hazards of vegan sausages. *The Telegraph*. June 11, 2024. Accessed October 11, 2025. https://www.telegraph.co.uk/health-fitness/nutrition/diet/vegan-sausages-vegetarian-health-hazards-heck-meat-free/

934 Whittaker R, Pickles K. Vegan fake meats are linked to increase in heart deaths, study suggests: experts say plant-based diets can boost health – but NOT if they are ultra-processed. *Daily Mail*. September 7, 2024. Accessed June 4, 2025. https://www.dailymail.co.uk/health/article-13182545/vegan-fake-meats-heart-deaths-study.html

935 Rauber F, Laura da Costa Louzada M, Chang K, et al. Implications of food ultra-processing on cardiovascular risk considering plant origin foods: an analysis of the UK Biobank cohort. *Lancet Reg Health Eur*. 2024;43:100948. doi: 10.1016/j.lanepe.2024.100948

936 Beslay M, Srour B, Méjean C, et al. Ultra-processed food intake in association with BMI change and risk of overweight and obesity: a prospective analysis of the French NutriNet-Santé cohort. *PLoS Med*. 2020;17(8):e1003256. doi: 10.1371/journal.pmed.1003256

937 Cordova R, Viallon V, Fontvieille E, et al. Consumption of ultra-processed foods and risk of multimorbidity of cancer and cardiometabolic diseases: a multinational cohort study. *Lancet Reg Health Eur*. 2023;35:100771. doi: 10.1016/j.lanepe.2023.100771

938 Cordova R, Viallon V, Fontvieille E, et al. Consumption of ultra-processed foods and risk of multimorbidity of cancer and cardiometabolic diseases: a multinational cohort study. *Lancet Reg Health Eur*. 2023;35:100771. doi: 10.1016/j.lanepe.2023.100771

939 Cordova R, Viallon V, Fontvieille E, et al. Consumption of ultra-processed foods and risk of multimorbidity of cancer and cardiometabolic diseases: a multinational cohort study. *Lancet Reg Health Eur*. 2023;35:100771. doi: 10.1016/j.lanepe.2023.100771

940 Visioli F, Del Rio D, Fogliano V, Marangoni F, Poli A. Ultra processed foods and cancer. *Lancet Reg Health Eur*. 2024;38:100863. doi: 10.1016/j.lanepe.2024.100863

941 Freisling H, Córdova R, Aune D, Wagner KH. Ultra processed foods and cancer—authors' reply. *Lancet Reg Health Eur*. 2024;38:100865. doi: 10.1016/j.lanepe.2024.100865

942 Dicken SJ, Dahm CC, Ibsen DB, et al. Food consumption by degree of food processing and risk of type 2 diabetes mellitus: a prospective cohort analysis of the European Prospective Investigation into Cancer and Nutrition (Epic). *Lancet Reg Health Eur.* 2024;46:101043.

943 Li C, Zhang Y, Zhang K, et al. Association between ultra-processed food consumption and leucocyte telomere length: a cross-sectional study of UK Biobank. *J Nutr.* 2024;154(10):3060–9. doi: 10.1016/j.tjnut.2024.05.001

944 Lousuebsakul-Matthews V, Thorpe DL, Knutsen R, Beeson WL, Fraser GE, Knutsen SF. Legumes and meat analogues consumption are associated with hip fracture risk independently of meat intake among Caucasian men and women: the Adventist Health Study-2. *Public Health Nutr.* 2014;17(10):2333–43. doi: 10.1017/S1368980013002693

945 Sabaté J, Wien M. Vegetarian diets and childhood obesity prevention. *Am J Clin Nutr.* 2010;91(5):1525S–9. doi: 10.3945/ajcn.2010.28701F

946 Jansen EC, Marín C, Mora-Plazas M, Villamor E. Higher childhood red meat intake frequency is associated with earlier age at menarche. *J Nutr.* 2015;146(4):792–8. doi: 10.3945/jn.115.226456

947 Kissinger DG, Sanchez A. The association of dietary factors with the age of menarche. *Nutr Res.* 1987;7(5):471–9. doi: 10.1016/S0271-5317(87)80003-9

948 Miller CA, Corbin KD, da Costa KA, et al. Effect of egg ingestion on trimethylamine-N-oxide production in humans: a randomized, controlled, dose-response study. *Am J Clin Nutr.* 2014;100(3):778–86.

949 Barnard ND, Long MB, Ferguson JM, Flores R, Kahleova H. Industry funding and cholesterol research: a systematic review. *Am J Lifestyle Med.* 2021;15(2):165–72.

950 Erlich MN, Ghidanac D, Blanco Mejia S, et al. A systematic review and meta-analysis of randomized trials of substituting soymilk for cow's milk and intermediate cardiometabolic outcomes: understanding the impact of dairy alternatives in the transition to plant-based diets on cardiometabolic health. *BMC Med.* 2024;22(1):336. doi: 10.1186/s12916-024-03524-7

951 Johnson AJ, Stevenson J, Pettit J, Jasthi B, Byhre T, Harnack L. Assessing the nutrient content of plant-based milk alternative products available in the United States. *J Acad Nutr Diet.* 2025;125(4):515–27.e8. doi: 10.1016/j.jand.2024.06.003

952 Drewnowski A, Henry CJ, Dwyer JT. Proposed nutrient standards for plant-based beverages intended as milk alternatives. *Front Nutr.* 2021;8:761442. doi: 10.3389/fnut.2021.761442

953 Khalil ZA, Herter-Aeberli I. Contribution of plant-based dairy and fish alternatives to iodine nutrition in the Swiss diet: a Swiss market survey. *Eur J Nutr.* 2024;63(5):1501–12. doi: 10.1007/s00394-024-03339-5

954 Ma W, He X, Braverman L. Iodine content in milk alternatives. *Thyroid.* 2016;26(9):1308–10. doi: 10.1089/thy.2016.0239

955 Khalil ZA, Herter-Aeberli I. Contribution of plant-based dairy and fish alternatives to iodine nutrition in the Swiss diet: a Swiss market survey. *Eur J Nutr.* 2024;63(5):1501–12. doi: 10.1007/s00394-024-03339-5

956 Shen P, Walker GD, Yuan Y, et al. Effects of soy and bovine milk beverages on enamel mineral content in a randomized, double-blind *in situ* clinical study. *J Dent.* 2019;88:103160. doi: 10.1016/j.jdent.2019.06.007

957   Huang Y, Thompson T, Wang Y, et al. Analysis of cariogenic potential of alternative milk beverages by *in vitro Streptococcus mutans* biofilm model and *ex vivo* caries model. *Arch Oral Biol.* 2019;105:52–8. doi: 10.1016/j.archoralbio.2019.05.033

958   Lee J, Townsend JA, Thompson T, et al. Analysis of the cariogenic potential of various almond milk beverages using a *Streptococcus mutans* biofilm model *in vitro. Caries Res.* 2018;52(1-2):51–7. doi: 10.1159/000479936

959   Dashper SG, Saion BN, Stacey MA, et al. Acidogenic potential of soy and bovine milk beverages. *J Dent.* 2012;40(9):736–41. doi: 10.1016/j.jdent.2012.05.004

960   Shen P, Walker GD, Yuan Y, et al. Effects of soy and bovine milk beverages on enamel mineral content in a randomized, double-blind *in situ* clinical study. *J Dent.* 2019;88:103160. doi: 10.1016/j.jdent.2019.06.007

961   Shkembi B, Huppertz T. Impact of dairy products and plant-based alternatives on dental health: food matrix effects. *Nutrients.* 2023;15(6):1469. doi: 10.3390/nu15061469

962   Messina M, Sievenpiper JL, Williamson P, Kiel J, Erdman JW. Perspective: soy-based meat and dairy alternatives, despite classification as ultra-processed foods, deliver high-quality nutrition on par with unprocessed or minimally processed animal-based counterparts. *Adv Nutr.* 2022;13(3):726–38. doi: 10.1093/advances/nmac026

963   Erlich MN, Ghidanac D, Blanco Mejia S, et al. A systematic review and meta-analysis of randomized trials of substituting soymilk for cow's milk and intermediate cardiometabolic outcomes: understanding the impact of dairy alternatives in the transition to plant-based diets on cardiometabolic health. *BMC Med.* 2024;22(1):336. doi: 10.1186/s12916-024-03524-7

964   Ference BA, Ginsberg HN, Graham I, et al. Low-density lipoproteins cause atherosclerotic cardiovascular disease. 1. Evidence from genetic, epidemiologic, and clinical studies. A consensus statement from the European Atherosclerosis Society Consensus Panel. *Eur Heart J.* 2017;38(32):2459–72. doi: 10.1093/eurheartj/ehx144

965   Springmann M. A multicriteria analysis of meat and milk alternatives from nutritional, health, environmental, and cost perspectives. *Proc Natl Acad Sci U S A.* 2024;121(50):e2319010121. doi: 10.1073/pnas.2319010121

966   Agricultural Research Service, United States Department of Agriculture. Beans, black, mature seeds, cooked, boiled, without salt. FoodData Central. April 2019. Accessed September 19, 2025. https://fdc.nal.usda.gov/food-details/173735/nutrients

967   Hosseinpour-Niazi S, Mirmiran P, Fallah-Ghohroudi A, Azizi F. Non-soya legume-based therapeutic lifestyle change diet reduces inflammatory status in diabetic patients: a randomised cross-over clinical trial. *Br J Nutr.* 2015;114(2):213–9. doi: 10.1017/S0007114515001725

968   Hosseinpour-Niazi S, Mirmiran P, Hedayati M, Azizi F. Substitution of red meat with legumes in the therapeutic lifestyle change diet based on dietary advice improves cardiometabolic risk factors in overweight type 2 diabetes patients: a cross-over randomized clinical trial. *Eur J Clin Nutr.* 2015;69(5):592–7. doi: 10.1038/ejcn.2014.228

969   Azadbakht L, Kimiagar M, Mehrabi Y, et al. Soy inclusion in the diet improves features of the metabolic syndrome: a randomized crossover study in postmenopausal women. *Am J Clin Nutr.* 2007;85(3):735–41. doi: 10.1093/ajcn/85.3.735

970   Messina M, Duncan AM, Glenn AJ, Mariotti F. Perspective: plant-based meat alternatives can help facilitate and maintain a lower animal to plant protein intake ratio. *Adv Nutr.* 2023;14(3):392–405. doi: 10.1016/j.advnut.2023.03.003

971 Hu FB, Otis BO, McCarthy G. Can plant-based meat alternatives be part of a healthy and sustainable diet? *JAMA*. 2019;322(16):1547–8. doi: 10.1001/jama.2019.13187

972 Springmann M. A multicriteria analysis of meat and milk alternatives from nutritional, health, environmental, and cost perspectives. *Proc Natl Acad Sci U S A*. 2024;121(50):e2319010121. doi: 10.1073/pnas.2319010121

973 Carroll L. Plant-based meat substitutes may be healthier for the heart than real meat, new analysis says. *NBC News*. June 26, 2024. Updated June 27, 2024. Accessed June 4, 2025. https://www.nbcnews.com/health/health-news/plant-based-meat-substitutes-may-healthier-heart-real-meat-new-analysis-rcna153456

974 Monteiro CA. Nutrition and health. The issue is not food, nor nutrients, so much as processing. *Public Health Nutr*. 2009;12(5):729–31. doi: 10.1017/S1368980009005291

975 Taylor C. Will the future forget about meat? *Mashable*. May 6, 2021. Accessed June 4, 2025. https://mashable.com/feature/dear-22nd-century-future-food-meat

976 Reynolds M. Fat, sugar, salt ... you've been thinking about food all wrong. *Wired*. February 22, 2023. Accessed June 4, 2025. https://www.wired.com/story/ultra-processed-foods

977 Bryant CJ. Plant-based animal product alternatives are healthier and more environmentally sustainable than animal products. *Future Foods*. 2022;6:100174. doi: 10.1016/j.fufo.2022.100174

978 Ketelings L, Benerink E, Havermans RC, Kremers SPJ, de Boer A. Fake meat or meat with benefits? How Dutch consumers perceive health and nutritional value of plant-based meat alternatives. *Appetite*. 2023;188:106616. doi: 10.1016/j.appet.2023.106616

979 Flint M, Bowles S, Lynn A, Paxman JR. Novel plant-based meat alternatives: future opportunities and health considerations. *Proc Nutr Soc*. 2023;82(3):370–85. doi: 10.1017/S0029665123000034

980 ZOE Editorial Staff. Is plant-based meat healthy? With Prof. Christopher Gardner. *ZOE*. June 12, 2024. Accessed June 4, 2025. https://zoe.com/learn/podcast-plant-based-meat-christopher-gardner

981 Barnard ND, Willett WC, Ding EL. The misuse of meta-analysis in nutrition research. *JAMA*. 2017;318(15):1435–6. doi: 10.1001/jama.2017.12083

982 Oldways. *Oldways Common Ground Consensus Statement on Healthy Eating*. November 19, 2015. Accessed June 4, 2025. https://oldwayspt.org/wp-content/uploads/2023/09/OW_CommonGround_Nov19.pdf

983 IARC Working Group on the Evaluation of Carcinogenic Risks to Humans. *Red Meat and Processed Meat*. International Agency for Research on Cancer; 2018. PMID: 29949327.

984 Office on Smoking and Health. *The Health Consequences of Involuntary Exposure to Tobacco Smoke: A Report of the Surgeon General*. U.S. Centers for Disease Control and Prevention; 2006. PMID: 20669524.

985 Pointke M, Pawelzik E. Plant-based alternative products: are they healthy alternatives? Micro- and macronutrients and nutritional scoring. *Nutrients*. 2022;14(3):601. doi: 10.3390/nu14030601

986 Taneri PE, Wehrli F, Roa-Díaz ZM, et al. Association between ultra-processed food intake and all-cause mortality: a systematic review and meta-analysis. *Am J Epidemiol*. 2022;191(7):1323–35. doi:10.1093/aje/kwac039

INDEX

Symbols

I

IGF-1 82, 83, 84
ileal brake 24
industrial pollutants 82
infant formula 46
inflammation 49, 60, 61, 72, 75, 84, 85, 89, 107, 109, 111
insulin resistance 69, 73, 74, 113
irritable bowel syndrome (IBS) 7, 61

J

junk food 4, 7, 8, 11, 29, 34, 37, 39, 106

K

kidney function 89, 107

L

LDL cholesterol 89, 93, 95, 96, 97, 98, 99, 107, 109
life expectancy 5, 35

M

meat methadone 113
methionine 82, 83
methylcellulose 59, 61, 77
microbial loads 80
microplastics 16, 66
mineral oils 16
mold toxins 86, 87
Monteiro, Carlos 3, 4, 49, 113, 114
mortality 5, 63, 73, 105, 109, 113, 115
mycoprotein 67, 69, 70, 87, 88, 90, 96

N

Neu5Gc 82, 85
nitrites 58, 59
nitrosamines 58
NOVA Classification System 3, 4, 31, 32, 33, 41, 42, 44, 45, 73
Nutrient Deficiency Era 1
Nutri-Score 52

O

obesity 1, 5, 7, 16, 23, 37, 73, 90, 103, 106
oxidative stress 49, 72, 73, 75, 84, 107

P

packaging chemicals 16, 66
parasites 78
phthalates 16, 17